THE OPEN UNIVERSITY

Science: A Second Level Course

COMPARATIVE PHYSIOLOGY

Unit 8   Hormones and the Reproductive Cycle

Unit 9   Hormones and Homeostasis: Blood Sugar and Blood Calcium

Unit 10 Hormones and Homeostasis: Osmoregulation and Excretion

Unit 11 Physiological Mechanisms and Physiological Evolution

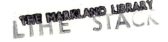
Prepared by the Course Team

The Open University Press

THE COMPARATIVE PHYSIOLOGY COURSE TEAM

M. E. Varley (*Course Team Chairman and General Editor*)
D. Adamson
H. Adamson (*Churchill Fellow*, 1971)
E. A. Bowers
N. R. Chalmers
R. Cordell
R. M. Holmes
S. W. Hurry
T. Laryea (*BBC*)
J. McCloy (*BBC*)
G. D. Moss
S. P. R. Rose
J. N. Thomas
R. Harding (*Course Assistant*)

The Open University Press
Walton Hall Bletchley Bucks

First published 1972

Designed by the Media Development Group of the Open University.

Printed in Great Britain by
Martin Cadbury Printing Group

SBN 335 02294 4

This text forms part of the correspondence element of an Open University Second Level Course. The complete list of units in the course is given at the end of this text.

For general availability of supporting material referred to in this text, please write to the Director of Marketing, The Open University, Walton Hall, Bletchley, Bucks.

Further information on Open University courses may be obtained from the Admissions Office, The Open University, P.O. Box 48, Bletchley, Bucks.

Hormones and the Reproductive Cycle
Unit 8

Contents

Table A

List of Scientific Terms, Concepts and Principles used in Unit 8

Taken as prerequisites			Introduced in these Units			
1 Assumed from general knowledge	**2** Introduced in previous Unit	Unit No.	**3** Developed in these Units	Page No.	**4** Developed in a later Unit	Unit No.
		S100				
parturition	stereoisomerism	10	hormone	7		
placenta	acetylcholine	18	neurendocrines	8		
uterus	adrenalin	18	neurohormones	8		
	endocrine gland	18	neurohumors	8		
	hormone	18	parahormones	8		
	hypothalamus	18	pheromone	8, 30		
			blastocyst	10		
			endometrium	10		
			Graafian follicle	10		
			implantation	10		
			menstrual cycle	10		
			ovulation	10		
			corpus luteum	11		
			oestrous cycle	11		
			colostrum	12		
			dioestrous	12		
			gestation	12		
			luteolysis	12		
			monoestrous	12		
			polyoestrous	12		
			pseudopregnancy	12		
			epididymis	14		
			seminiferous tubules	14		
			androgen, testosterone	16		
			oestrogen	16		
			steroids	16		
			oestradiol	17		
			follicle stimulating hormone (FSH)	19		
			gonadotrophin	19		
			hypophysectomy	20		
			hypothalamus	20		
			luteinizing hormone (LH)	20		
			synergism	20		
			progesterone	21		
			antagonism	22		
			FSH/LH–RH	24		
			prostaglandin	24		
			Leydig cells	25		
			Sertoli cells	25		
			pampiniform plexus	26		
			induced ovulation	27		
			spontaneous ovulation	27		
			short and long day breeders	29		
			genotypic and phenotypic sex	30		
			free-martin	32		
			genital ridge	32		

Objectives (*Units 8 and 9*)

After reading these Units you should be able to:

1 Define, recognize the best definitions of or put into proper context the terms and principles included in Table A.

2 Make valid generalizations on the interrelation of nervous and hormonal systems in achieving homeostasis or controlled variation in physiological systems.

3 Cite at least four examples of the relationship between the nervous system and the hormonal regulation of a physiologically important factor.

4 Show an understanding of various aspects of the hormonal control of the reproductive cycle of the mammal by making predictions as to the probable outcome of suggested experimental procedures.

5 Distinguish between well-founded and unfounded hypotheses as to the probable mechanisms regulating the following: the onset of the oestrous cycle, ovulation, the duration of the oestrous cycle, cyclical changes in the genital tract, spermatogenesis, level of blood calcium, the level of blood sugar.

6 Give examples of the following: two or more different hormones acting synergistically in the production of a physiological or anatomical effect; two hormones acting antagonistically in the production of a physiological effect; two hormones which act synergistically on one target organ but antagonistically on another; a negative feedback relationship between two hormones which does not result in homeostasis.

7 Give examples of the following:
(a) Hormones which act antagonistically to achieve the homeostasis of a substance in the blood stream.
(b) Different hormones which tend to have similar effects on the homeostasis of substances in the blood stream.

8 Distinguish different types of antagonistic relationships between hormones involved in homeostatic mechanisms, including direct feedback effects and effects dependent on the level of a third factor.

9 Show an understanding of the mechanisms involved in the maintenance of blood sugar levels in vertebrates (particularly mammals) by making, or selecting, predictions of the outcome of various experimental procedures.

10 Show an understanding of the mechanisms involved in the maintenance of blood calcium levels in mammals by making or selecting, predictions as to the outcome of various experimental procedures.

Study Guide

Unit 8 is the first of a group of three Units (8, 9 and 10) which form a block dealing with hormones.

You should recall that hormones are discussed in S100,* Unit 18, and may find it helpful to re-read that Unit before starting on this one.

Hormones are discussed and classified in Section 8.1, laying the foundation for the studies of integrative action of hormones that follow.

The rest of the Unit is largely concerned with reproductive organs (described in Section 8.2), reproductive cycles and the hormones that regulate them (8.3) and how these cycles are related to changes in external environment (8.4). Female mammal cycles are studied in detail because much information is available about them and they are remarkably regular and predictable. The reproduction of male mammals is much less cyclical, and you could omit study of this (Section 8.3.5) if you are short of time. Other vertebrates are referred to occasionally.

The Unit concludes with a short section on sex determination (8.5) but you could omit it if short of time. It illustrates one-off effects of sex hormones.

There is no prescribed set book for this Unit.

The Home Experiment is a study of ferret reproduction as revealed by microscope sections E_1 and E_2 and photographs.

You are advised not to attempt this investigation until you have completed all the work described in the Home Experiment Notes of Unit 4 and have looked at slides A, B and C. Although it is officially assigned to Unit 8 because it concerns reproduction, this work represents the final instalment of your assignment on animal histology. There is no need for you to do it until near the end of this Course.

* *The Open University (1971) S100* Science: A Foundation Course, *The Open University Press.*

8.0 Introduction to Units 8, 9 and 10

Living organisms exhibit a number of characteristics, among which are nutrition, respiration, growth, internal co-ordination, sensitivity to the environment, and reproduction. In Units 2–6 we considered some of the ways in which organisms obtain from the environment the raw materials needed for respiration, growth and reproduction; also some details of how they are transported within the organism. In Unit 7 we considered growth, and some of the factors regulating it. In Units 8, 9 and 10 we are going to look at different means by which internal co-ordination is achieved in animals, particularly those involving hormones. By selecting the examples carefully we hope to be able to make some valid generalizations about co-ordination, while at the same time giving you more information on some of the processes of reproduction, metabolism and regulation which take place in animals.

Although in this book there are four Units, three are on a single major theme—internal co-ordination by means of hormones—and you should view them as different illustrations of this theme.

8.1 Hormones

Study Comment

In this Section hormones are discussed and classified. It is important that you should read this carefully and note the four broad types of integration that may result from hormone action.

You will know from S100, Unit 18, and perhaps also from other sources, that the two 'systems' responsible for physiological co-ordination are the nervous and endocrine systems. For a detailed study of nervous co-ordination you must follow the parallel course to this one, *Biological Bases of Behaviour**; here we consider mainly endocrine control—though the two systems are not really separable.

You have already encountered the word 'hormone' in S100, Unit 18 and again in Units 4 and 7 of this Course. In S100, Unit 18, we defined a hormone as the secretion of a gland, released into the blood plasma and thus carried to a 'target' organ on which it exerts its effect.

In Unit 4 we discussed some of the hormones involved in the co-ordination of digestion, and simply said that they were produced by secretory cells in the gut wall. In Unit 7 we talked of plant growth substances, and said that in animals these would be called growth hormones.

The traditional definition of a hormone is close to the one we gave you in S100, except that where we defined a 'gland' as 'a collection of secretory cells', the traditional view is that it is a 'discrete, circumscribed, specialized structure, clearly recognizable as either endocrine or ductless'. You will see that both our original definition and the traditional one would automatically exclude the plant growth substances. Also excluded would be the adrenalin released at the termination of the post-ganglionic fibres of the sympathetic nervous system; yet the adrenalin released by the adrenal medulla, an obvious endocrine gland, would be included. However, the tissues of the adrenal medulla are in fact nervous in origin—they are highly modified post-ganglionic sympathetic nerve fibres, specialized for adrenalin secretion rather than nervous conduction. This makes the distinction look a little arbitrary. More confusing than this, however, is the classification of the substances produced by functional nerve cells, released into the blood stream and acting on target organs; you have already encountered the TRF (thyrotrophin releasing factor) secreted by the hypothalamus into the portal venous system of the pituitary (S100, Unit 18). There are in addition a number of other substances produced by nerve cells and released into the general circulation in many invertebrates and all vertebrates; for example, the secretions of the posterior lobe of the pituitary (the 'neurohypophysis'), mentioned in

---

* *The Open University (1972) SDT 286 Biological Bases of Behaviour (BBB) A Second Level Course, The Open University Press.*

7

Unit 10. If none of these is to be considered a hormone, then clearly the term loses much of its usefulness.

The disadvantage of throwing the definition wide open to include *any* product of a cell or group of cells which affects the metabolism or the action of other organs is that it will then include such things as the CO_2 produced by respiration, and once again the term loses its usefulness.

The best approach is probably to compromise, taking the traditional definition as the starting-point; then widening it to include the products of neurosecretory cells, calling them *neurohormones* or *neuroendocrines*. These can be distinguished from the acetylcholine or adrenalin produced at the nerve terminations by calling these *neurohumors*; the distinction is arbitrary but useful.

neurohormones
neuroendocrines
neurohumors

There are whole groups of chemicals, released by individual cells in response to damage or attack, or in some cases anoxia, which may be of great importance in producing appropriate responses by other parts of the body. There are also chemical responses to certain antigens, which play a part in the immune reactions of the body. These substances, and many others, are probably best described as *parahormones*, and could be considered as the animal equivalents of the plant growth substances.

parahormones

Finally, there are some substances which could be reasonably classed as hormones, but for the fact that they are transmitted from one individual to another across the environment. They may produce either behavioural or endocrine changes in the recipient. The substance may be air-borne, as with some sex attractants, or eaten, as with the 9-ketodecanoic acid in the 'queen substance' produced by the queen bee and eaten by the workers. At the moment, this type of chemical messenger is called a *pheromone*—and we will discuss them further in this Unit.

pheromone

Hormones characteristically act by producing a change in the rate of the activity of the target tissues, thus, for example, selectively changing the rate at which a substance is secreted into, or absorbed from, the blood. This may lead to a number of things, from the differential growth of an organ in the body to ovulation or a change in body temperature.

It is possible to generalize about hormone action at the physiological level, and say that there are four broad types of integration produced by the action of what we can call hormones 'proper': (1) 'one off' situations, permanent or transient changes produced by the secretion of a hormone at a particular time; (2) a complicated, sequential series of responses, one following the other until some conclusion is reached—in short, a cycle which then may or may not be immediately repeated; (3) a 'constant level' or homeostatic situation, where potential change is resisted; (4) the integration of one of the above actions with the outside environment, i.e. timing a cycle or shifting the 'constant level'.

four types of hormonal integration

QUESTION   Can you, from your general knowledge or the work you have done to date, think of examples of these four types of integration?

ANSWER   1   Action of adrenalin released in response to sudden stress; also you will be aware of the development of the 'secondary sexual characteristics', many of which are dependent on the secretion of 'male' or 'female' hormones at a particular stage of development.

2   We have not considered clear examples of the co-ordination of cycles, though again you may be aware of reproductive cycles.

3   Regulation of the metabolic rate by thyroxin.

4   We have not considered this in detail: adrenalin is released in response to environmental factors, but this is directly under nervous control. You may know, however, that the level of thyroxin secretion, and thus the metabolic rate, varies between summer and winter. You will also know that many animals are only able to reproduce at certain times of year.

Classifying hormone actions in this way is of course quite arbitrary in that it does not necessarily imply real differences in the effects at a cellular level—indeed in some cases we may be considering different effects of the same hormones. You may well find examples of hormone action that do not really fit in any of the above categories. However, the advantage of looking at them in this way is that it does emphasize how widely different the physiological effects may be, even where at a biochemical level the actions are closely similar.

One reason for studying vertebrate reproductive cycles, apart from their obvious intrinsic interest to a biologist, is that they provide extremely clear examples of integration by hormones, particularly of the first, second and fourth types mentioned above.

8.2 Mammalian Reproductive Cycles

Study Comment

This Section gives basic information about the reproductive organs of mammals and the cycles of events in mature females and males. If you already know about these, you can omit this Section. Physiological interpretations in later Sections assume knowledge of information given here.

Mammalian reproductive hormones have been studied in great detail over the last thirty years or so, and it is for this reason that we shall concentrate largely on mammals with occasional references to other vertebrates and invertebrates. Although there is now quite a lot of information about the occurrence of different sex hormones in other vertebrates, particularly birds, much of what is believed about their action in fact arises by extrapolation from the mammalian work.

Before considering the role of hormones, we will give a brief and very simple account of the events of the reproductive cycle in placental mammals, with particular reference to man. If you are familiar with these events, move on to Section 8.3.

In most vertebrates, and all mammals, there are two distinct sexes, male and female. Sex reversal occasionally occurs in fish; some teleosts are truly hermaphrodite and able to produce both eggs and sperm at the same time.

8.2.1 Female mammals

A female placental mammal is equipped with paired *ovaries*, in which the eggs are produced, and *oviducts* (*Fallopian tubes*), with funnels (*fimbria*) applied closely to the ovaries; these tubes lead to a *uterus* or womb, which may be single, as in primates (Fig. 1), double as in rats, or a compromise as in the pig, where there are two very distinct 'horns' of the uterus but a small common 'body' and only one *cervix*. In rats and mice there are two quite separate cervices opening into the *vagina*, so that the uteri are quite separate. The vagina opens externally, guarded by the *vulva*. In the marsupial mammals (S100, Unit 21) there are two quite separate tracts, with two vaginae, and the male has an appropriately cleft penis.

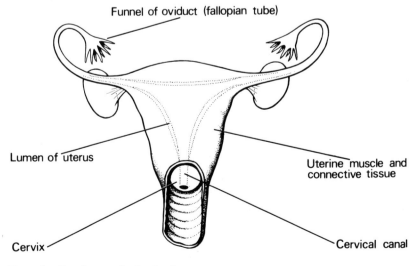

Funnel of oviduct (fallopian tube)

Lumen of uterus

Uterine muscle and connective tissue

Cervix

Cervical canal

Figure 1 Female reproductive tract.

9

Within the ovaries (Fig. 2) there are *primordial follicles*, containing the cells which give rise to the egg and its surrounding membranes; they are present from birth in large numbers (many thousands) and it is possible that no new ones are produced during post-natal development. Certainly there are more present at birth than can ever ripen and be shed.

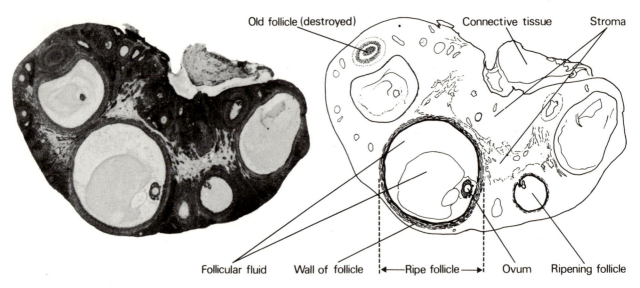

Old follicle (destroyed) Connective tissue Stroma

Follicular fluid   Wall of follicle |←— Ripe follicle —→| Ovum   Ripening follicle

Figure 2   Very low power photomicrograph of transverse section of an ovary showing follicles (with related diagram).

These primordial follicles ripen into large 'Graafian follicles' (Fig. 2) and these burst to release the egg, a process called *ovulation*. The egg is, of course, produced by meiosis, and is therefore haploid. In primates, including women, generally only one follicle ovulates at a time, though sometimes several may ripen together, shedding more than one egg. Whether, in women, the two ovaries alternate, one shedding an egg one month and the other the next, as is commonly believed, is not determined. Certainly women with only one ovary can ovulate each month.

ovulation

Many mammals regularly produce a number of eggs from each ovary at each ovulation, for example the dog, cat, pig, ferret, rabbit and many others. The elephant shrew probably takes pride of place, shedding over one hundred eggs per ovulation. An alternative system is shown by the nine-banded armadillo; like the primates, it sheds a single egg, but after it is fertilized the zygote divides into four, giving rise to identical quadruplets.

After ovulation the egg or eggs pass down the Fallopian tube, a process which generally takes a couple of days in women; fertilization by the spermatozoa from the male takes place in the Fallopian tubes, after which the egg begins to divide to form a *blastocyst*. You can see ovulation and the movement of the egg into the tube on the television programme for this Unit.

blastocyst

Whether or not a fertilized egg implants in the uterus seems to depend to a large extent on the state of the *endometrium* (epithelial lining) of the uterus; for a certain limited period of time after ovulation the endometrium is highly receptive to anything lying on it. It will grow round and to some extent nourish the blastocyst or, for that matter, in some species such as the guinea pig, pieces of thread, glass balls or foreign tissue as well if you put them there at the right time.

endometrium

However, the blastocyst itself certainly plays an active part in implantation—it will attach itself to non-endometrial surfaces if it is misplaced, for example; later on, when it is well implanted, it attacks the maternal epithelial tissue as a normal part of placenta formation. It is not clear why only a few of the blastocysts implant in those species which shed many eggs at a time. In some species, such as the rabbit and the pig, it is common to find some early embryos being reabsorbed by the mother, that is to say, more blastocysts implant than are carried through to term. A number of species show delayed implantation (Section 8.4.3), the fertilized blastocyst remaining unattached for varying periods.

In women, ovulation takes place every 28 days or so, from puberty (usually from 12–14) until menopause (45–50). This cycle is called the *menstrual cycle* in

menstrual cycle

10

women and the other primates simply because there is visible bleeding (or *menstruation*) at the end of it. In mammals generally, the cycle is called the *oestrous cycle*, because most mammals show oestrous or 'heat' at about the time of ovulation becoming receptive to the advances of the male. (This effect is not marked in human females who may be receptive at any stage of the cycle, though there is a small change in body temperature at the time of ovulation.) We shall use the term 'oestrous cycle' for all mammals.

The events of the cycle show a high degree of co-ordination, an analysis of which is a major part of this Unit. The follicle or follicles develop in the ovary for the first 12–15 days of the human cycle (taking day 1 of the new cycle as the *first day of menstruation*). From the end of menstruation, say day 4, the endometrium begins to build up and become vascularized. (You will work out in detail what some of these changes are for yourselves in the investigation on the ferret associated with this Unit.) After ovulation, further build-up of the endometrium takes place, and in the ovary the ruptured follicle develops into a solid secretory body (Figs. 3 and 4) called the *corpus luteum*.

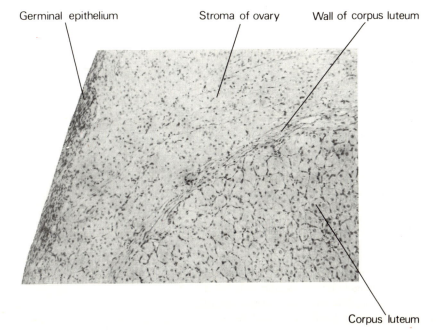

Corpora lutea

Immature follicles

Germinal epithelium   Stroma of ovary   Wall of corpus luteum

Corpus luteum

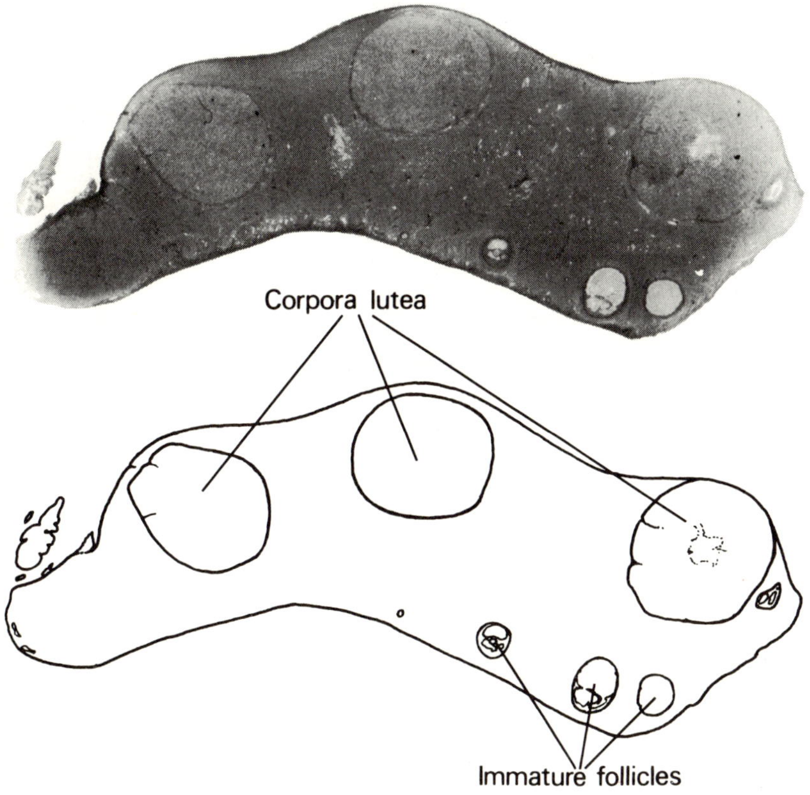

Figure 3   Very low power photomicrograph of longitudinal section of an ovary showing ripe corpora lutea (with related diagram).

Figure 4   Medium power photomicrograph showing upper edge of a corpus luteum and germinal epithelium of the ovary.

If fertilization and implantation occur, the corpus luteum persists, in some species throughout pregnancy, in others only through the early stages. The corpus luteum will also persist if the animal is *pseudopregnant*, that is, it is behaving physiologically as if it were pregnant when it is not. Such a state occurs quite commonly in animals such as the rat, rabbit and ferret (see Section 8.4.3 and Home Experiment).

pseudopregnancy

Normally when pregnancy does not occur, the corpus luteum is destroyed (*luteolysis*). In women, this will be about 13 days after ovulation. Following this, the endometrium begins to break up, shedding blood, epithelium, capillaries and other tissue into the lumen of the uterus; most of this escapes through the cervix and appears as the menstrual flow, marking day 1 of the new cycle. The duration of one cycle varies with the species. In mice it may be three days or five days depending on the genetic strain. In sheep it is sixteen days. A number of mammals are said to be *polyoestrous*, that is to say they have many oestrous cycles per year. Some polyoestrous animals, including women, the laboratory rat, mouse and the guinea pig, cycle continuously. Others have a series of sequential cycles through a limited breeding season—this is true of sheep, and many deer. Then there are *dioestrous* mammals, having just two heats a year (such as the bitch), and *monoestrous* ones with a single heat (these include the silver fox and some martens (Fig. 5)). In most cases these breeding seasons, whether they contain a single oestrous or many, are correlated with changes in the environment, such as variations in the food supply or temperature. Since the time at which food or temperature may be critical for the survival of the young may be as much as months away from the time of ovulation and mating, the influence will not be a direct one. For example, an autumn mating of ewes in Britain will give lambing in January or February and allow the lambs to be weaned on to spring grass and have the whole summer to grow. Clearly it is not spring conditions which directly determine the timing of oestrous.

luteolysis

polyoestrous

dioestrous and monoestrous mammals

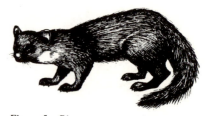

Figure 5   Pine marten.

When implantation and pregnancy occur, the corpus luteum persists as mentioned above, and further development of the endometrium continues for some time. A complex placenta is formed, starting from the point of implantation. It is made up of maternal tissue from the endometrium and tissue from the developing embryo. The function of the placenta is primarily to provide an exchange network between the embryo's blood system and the mother's without allowing the two blood systems actually to mix.

placenta

ITQ 1   Suggest reasons why allowing the mother's blood to flow through the embryo might be undesirable?

Read the answer to ITQ 1 (p. 35).

Respiratory gases can be exchanged through the placenta as well as food and nitrogenous waste. The placenta has also been shown to be an important source of hormones, particularly in those mammals where the corpus luteum does not persist throughout pregnancy.

In the second half of the oestrous cycle there is also some growth of mammary tissue, an effect which increases very much during pregnancy. In women, where mammary development occurs at puberty (the glands presumably being sustained to some extent by the continuous cycling), the increase is less marked. In many 'seasonal' mammals, however, the non-pregnant animal has scarcely any gland, as development occurs throughout the pregnancy. In all mammals, 'colostrum' (a clear proteinous secretion rather similar to milk) is secreted towards the end of the pregnancy, as is milk within a short time of the birth of the young.

mammary tissue

The duration of pregnancy (the *gestation* period) varies from mammal to mammal depending mainly on two factors: the actual size to which the foetus grows and the stage of development it reaches before it is born. Thus the laboratory rat and the hamster, animals of roughly similar size, have gestation periods of 21 and 18 days respectively; the guinea pig, again of comparable size, has a gestation period of 68 days. The reason for the difference lies in the stage of development reached by the young at the end of the period. Rats and hamsters

gestation period

have small, naked young with their eyes still closed; guinea pigs are born active, fully furred and with their eyes open, able to fend for themselves to quite a large extent. Table 1 below gives data on some selected mammals. You are not expected to memorize this Table but you may find the information useful.

Table 1

Species	Oestrous cycle (days)	Average gestation period (days)	Litter size (average)
European hedgehog	— (monoestrous)	34–49	5
European bat (*Vespertilio murinus*)	—	50	1
Rhesus monkey	28 ⎤ (polyoestrous continuous)	164	1–2
Chimpanzee	34 ⎬	237	1–2
Woman	28 ⎦	280	1–2
Armadillo, Nine-banded (*Dasypus novemcinctus*)	—	150	4
Indian elephant	(polyoestrous)	623	1–2
Blue whale	—	365	1–2
Domestic pig	21 (polyoestrous continuous)	113	6–11
Wild pig (*Sus cristatus*)		120	4–6
Domestic cattle	21 (polyoestrous almost continuous)	282	1–2
Domestic sheep	17 (polyoestrous seasonal)	150	1–6
Bighorn sheep (*Ovis canadensis*)		180	1
Ferret	none (see p. 27)	42	9
Domestic cat	15–21	63	4
Domestic rabbit	none (see p. 27)	31	6 (range 1–13)
Laboratory rat	4–6	21	7–9
Golden hamster	4	18	6
Guinea pig	$16\frac{1}{2}$	68	3
Laboratory mouse	5	19	6
Shrew (*Sorex araneus*)	—	15	7

The gestation period of a particular species (at least within a strain of that species) is normally very constant, varying between individuals by only 5–10 per cent. Thus the range of gestation periods in the Indian elephant is only 607 ± 41 days, in women 270 ± 10 days. The precision of the timing of this process has aroused much interest in recent years. It is not known precisely what initiates the start of the birth process (*parturition*), although a number of factors are known to play a part.

parturition

8.2.2 Male mammals

The male reproductive system is rather simpler than that of the female, as befits its more modest role. All male mammals have an intromittent organ, the *penis*, the evolution of mammals has been primarily terrestrial and embryonic development is internal; the transfer of delicate spermatozoa into the female vagina calls for a specific organ. The organ is erectile, and in some members of the Ursidae (bears) and Mustelidae (stoat, otters, badgers) it is supported by a small skeletal element. The *urethra*, the tube running through the penis, is common to both the urinary and genital systems as it leads directly to the bladder. Opening into the urethra a little below the bladder are the two *vasa deferentia* (singular: *vas deferens*) which carry sperm from the testes; also opening into it are ducts from Cowper's gland and the prostate gland, both important in the production of the seminal fluid. Seminal vesicles open into each vas deferens before they reach the urethra.

The testes are made up of coiled *seminiferous tubules*, the epithelial linings of which produce the sperm (Fig. 6). Between the tubules are connective tissues and the *Leydig cells* (or *interstitial tissue of the testis*) which are secretory (Fig. 7). Sperm is collected in a coiled tube attached to the testis, the *epididymis*, where it is stored until it is ejaculated in mating. The walls of the epididymis are contractile and move the sperm quite quickly, in the early stages of mating, to a segment of the vas deferens which runs into the urethra; this segment, called the ejaculatory duct, is very muscular and provides the main impetus for ejaculation, although there may be peristaltic movements of other ducts also.

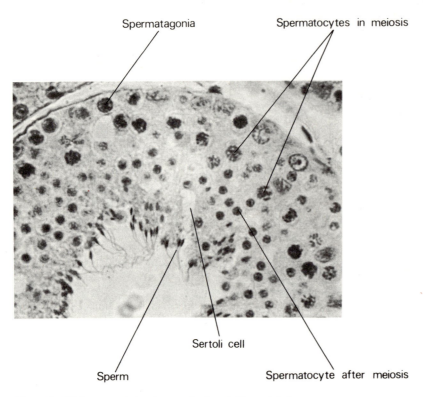

Figure 6   High power photomicrograph of seminiferous tubules.

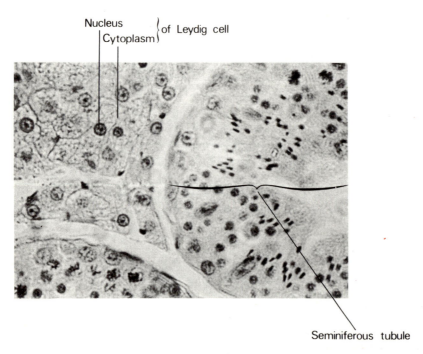

Figure 7   High power photomicrograph of seminiferous tubules and Leydig cells.

In most mammals the testes descend from the abdominal cavity into an external sac, the *scrotum*, apparently with the advantage that they are 1–3°C cooler than

scrotum

14

the internal organs; a temperature-dependent reflex governs a limited amount of movement of the scrotum and the testes themselves. In most mammals, spermatogenesis is prevented if the testes do not descend or are kept at full body temperature by other means.

Seasonal breeders may retract the inactive testes into the body cavity out of season, and a few species, including the whale, seal, elephant and rhinoceros retain them in the body cavity permanently.

There is no evidence of any cycle comparable to the oestrous cycle of the female, though there is a fairly lengthy cycle of sperm manufacture, which seems to occur about five times a year; however, this is not easy to detect, as it does not show in variations of the sperm count or in any other practical way. As we implied above, species which are seasonal breeders have active testes only in the breeding season, and only show mating behaviour at this time. Furthermore, **seasonal changes** there may be changes in appearance associated with the onset of the breeding season, e.g. growth of antlers in stags. (Birds show this even more clearly in their plumage changes.)

8.2.3 Comment

You will realize, even from the extremely brief descriptions in this Section, that literally dozens of questions arise as to how these processes are initiated, regulated and co-ordinated. Some of these can be answered with reasonable assurance, but many cannot. There is a lot of information now available, but it does not all fit into a clear picture. Furthermore, the mammalian reproductive system is unusual in comparison to the other systems, such as the nervous or circulatory systems, in that there is great variation from species to species. Much confusion in the past has arisen from apparently conflicting generalizations, the truth eventually emerging as 'a' in the rat and 'b' in the monkey. Man and the usual laboratory animals have been the source of most of the information, though a lot is now known of the reproductive physiology of domestic animals, particularly sheep, cattle and goats.

Finally, this is a field in which the old adage, 'he who simplifies simply lies', is all too true. Fortunately, we are not trying to present a comprehensive survey of reproductive physiology—that would take a minimum of a year's full-time study—we are trying to demonstrate some principles of hormone action and describe something of reproduction at the same time. Thus we hope to avoid lying, or even trivializing the subject too much, by ignoring much of it.

8.3 Co-ordination of the Reproductive Cycle

Study Comment

This Section discusses the hormonal control of reproductive cycles, especially those of female mammals. You need not remember the detailed chemical structures of the hormones. You should try to understand how the many hormones involved are integrated leading to cyclical changes and the relevance of this to contraception. If you are short of time, omit the male reproductive cycle (Section 8.3.5).

8.3.1 The steroid hormones

It has been known since classical times that much of the reproductive and 'sexual' nature of man and other animals depended on something produced by the ovaries of the female and the testes of the male. If the ovaries were removed, reproduction became impossible; if they were removed before puberty, the secondary sexual characteristics (mammary glands, enlarged vulva and in the case of women, deposition of subcutaneous fat) did not appear. Castration has been practised for as long as there have been records, with purposes ranging from the production of shrill voices to good beef; again both primary and secondary sexual characteristics were known to be affected.

Early research showed that much of the lost function could be restored to spayed or castrated animals by injecting extracts of ovaries or testes, and that an intact animal not on heat could be brought on heat by injection of the appropriate extract. In the case of females, this substance was therefore described as *oestrogen* or *oestrogenic*, meaning 'generating heat'. The extraction from the testes was called *androgen* or *androgenic*, 'generating maleness'.

The situation, of course, is now known to be vastly more complicated than this, but these hormones, oestrogen and androgen, can be identified as members of a group of substances known as steroids, and of the greatest importance to the body.

The steroids, which include substances such as cholesterol, found throughout the body, as well as the steroid hormones from the adrenal cortex, ovary, testis and placenta, share a common basic structure—the steroid nucleus.

Written in full, it has the structural formula shown in Figure 8, but it is normally abbreviated to the form shown in Figure 9.

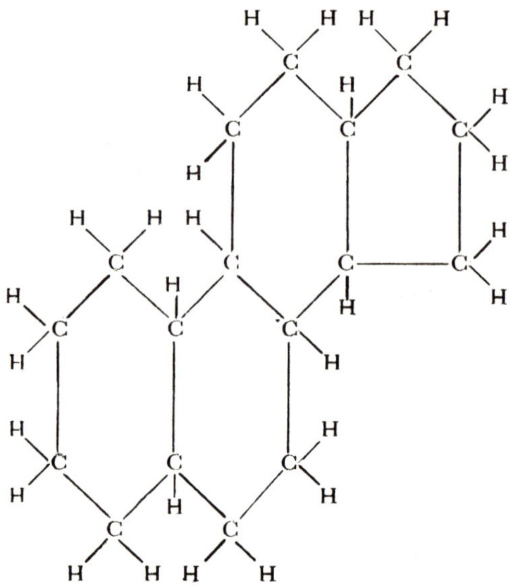

Figure 8   *Steroid nucleus (written in full).*

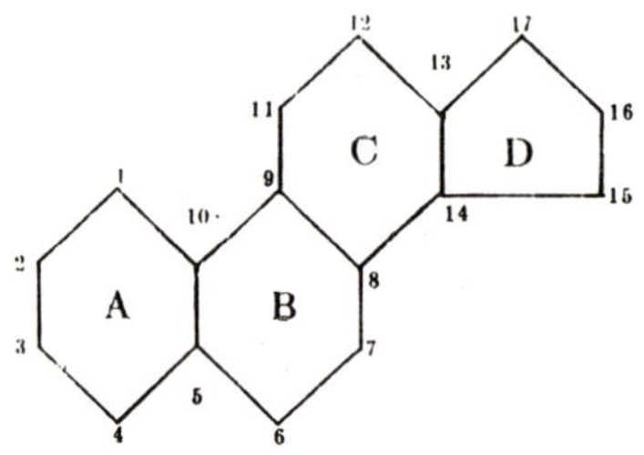

Figure 9   Steroid nucleus (normal abbreviation).

The carbon atoms are numbered as above, so that it is simple to describe the location of a particular side chain, by naming the carbon to which it is attached. The stereo-isomerism is described by calling groups which are 'cis' to a reference point, β, and those which are 'trans', α. Steroid molecules can therefore be named systematically in a way that describes them; they can also be given trivial names which are far easier to remember but tell you nothing of the molecule. Since in this Course it is not necessary to know details of the molecule, we will adopt the latter practice.

There are three generalizations about steroid hormones that you should remember, particularly if you do some reading on your own.

1   Small changes in the side chains may mean profound changes in the physiological effect. For example, the replacement of an —OH group by $=O$ on the 3C position is the main difference between oestradiol (an oestrogen from the ovary) and testosterone (an androgen from the testis), as shown in Figure 10.

2   One hormone is likely to be manufactured from another in the secretory cell, as they mostly originate from the same substances. If the gland is analysed it may yield many steroids that are in fact only metabolic precursors of the ones released. At least 40 steroids can be found in the adrenal cortex, but this does not mean they all have any physiological significance.

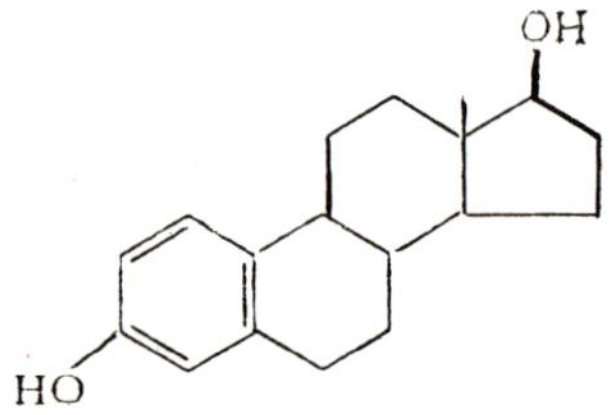

1,3,5(10)-oestratriene-3,17β-diol
(oestradiol-17β, from ovary)

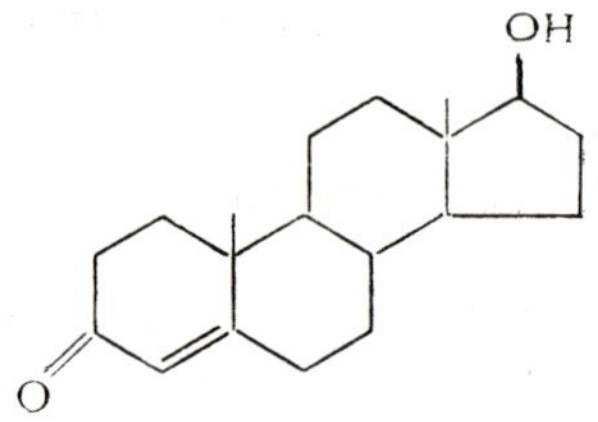

17β-hydroxy-4-androsten-3-one
(Testosterone, from testis)

Figure 10   *Formulae of oestradiol and testosterone.*

16

3   In practice, you will hear of steroids from three main sources: those occurring in the body; those which have been altered in the liver and found in the urine (where they are much easier to measure than in the blood); and the man-made synthetics. For the moment, try to think only in terms of the first group, though the others will be mentioned.

8.3.2   The female cycle

The evidence is that for the first half of the oestrous cycle, oestrogen, in particular oestradiol, is the dominant product of the ovary. The first question is: where in the ovary is it produced? The second: what regulates it?

oestradiol

QUESTION   Look at Figures 2, 11 and 12, photomicrographs of the ovary in the latter part of the pre-ovulatory phase of the oestrous cycle. You are asked to guess which cells you think are most likely to be the main source of the oestradiol. Recall what you know of the appearance of the nuclei of actively secreting cells from the histology investigations started as the Home Experiment for Unit 4.

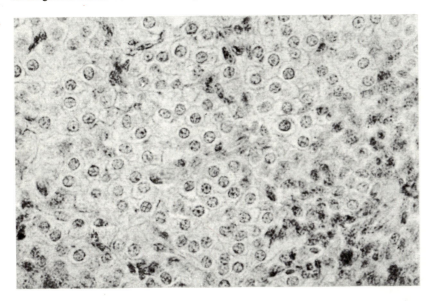

Figure 11   *High power photomicrograph of stroma of ovary.*

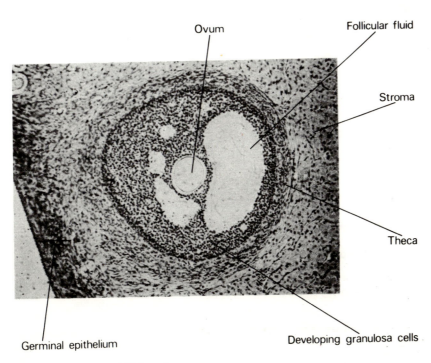

Figure 12   *Immature follicle and stroma.*

ANSWER You have probably guessed wrongly, according to the generally accepted view. The main 'background' tissue of the ovary, the *stroma*, seems a likely candidate. There is a lot of it, the cells are large and have large, round, pale nuclei; you may see that there are a lot of capillaries draining it (recognizable by their endothelial nuclei). However it is generally believed that the granulosa cells lining the inside of the follicles are the primary source (Figs. 13 and 14) and that the effective oestrogen is, in fact, follicular oestrogen.

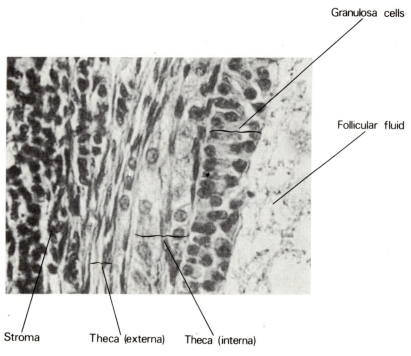

Figure 13 *High power photomicrograph of wall of mature follicle.*

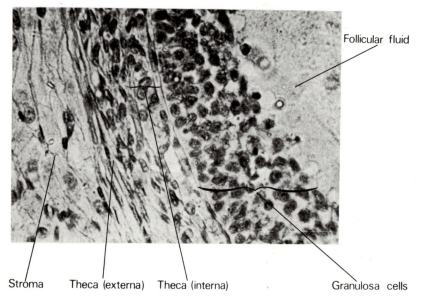

Figure 14 *High power photomicrograph of wall of immature follicle.*

The follicles are believed to be the source of oestrogen because:

1   The follicles can be seen to be growing in step with the level of blood oestradiol, during the first part of the cycle, and to fall sharply at the time they rupture (Fig. 15).

2   The fluid in the follicles has been sampled and contains a very strong concentration of oestradiol.

3   When the follicles were destroyed by X-rays, the output of oestradiol fell sharply.

18

4   The administration of hormones which increase follicle size and growth also increases blood oestradiol.

However, in spite of this evidence, it would not hurt to keep an open mind as to the main source of cyclical oestrogen. The granulosa cells do not constitute a great volume, and they are encased in the *theca externa* of the follicles, which is not very vascular, so the follicles do not seem at first sight to be the ideal of an endocrine gland (Figs. 13 and 14). The high concentration of oestradiol in the follicular fluid could be because it cannot escape rapidly. (Were the main source of oestradiol in the blood to be the stroma, the accumulation in those cells would not be expected to rise very high, because of their extensive blood supply.) Verification, or otherwise, of the long accepted view should be available soon.

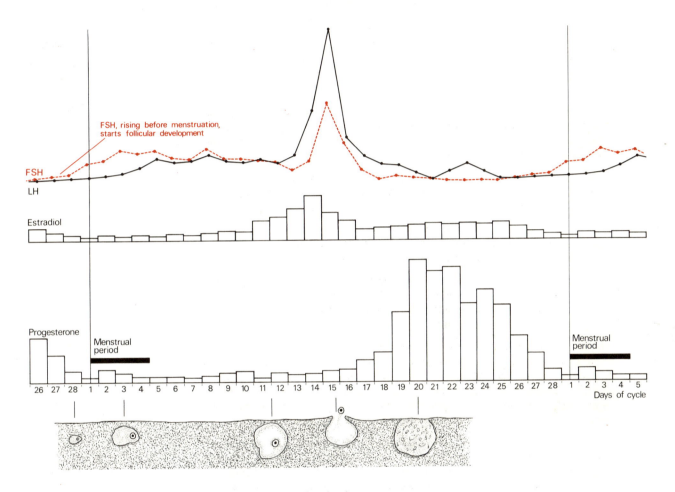

Figure 15   *Gonadotrophin/steroid levels during the menstrual cycle of a woman.*

If we accept the ripening follicles as the source of the oestradiol, the question remains: what causes them to ripen? From what we have said of the reproductive cycle, and what you know of physiological regulation, it is unlikely that follicular growth is spontaneous.

If the pituitary is removed, the follicles do not ripen; they recede and atrophy. Blood oestradiol falls to a very low, continuous 'base-line' level.

What does this suggest to you as a control mechanism? Recall thyroxin, S100, Unit 18.

It suggests some type of feedback mechanism with a pituitary hormone.

Where does this system differ from the thyroxin control system?

The negative feedback system regulated thyroxin at a steady state—homeostasis. Oestradiol levels are not steady—they rise and then fall.

Follicle growth and oestrogen production are regulated by the pituitary hormone known as Follicle Stimulating Hormone (FSH). It is not a steroid, it is a glyco-protein, one of a small group of pituitary hormones called gonadotrophins.

FSH

gonadotrophins

19

These are the so-called 'fertility drugs', and because of the variation in sensitivity between individuals, when administered artificially they may sometimes have the unfortunate effect of ripening many follicles instead of just one or two. It is very difficult to measure the levels of these hormones, it must usually be done by 'bio-assay' rather than by physical measurement. The sample is injected into an animal which has had its pituitary removed, and the extent to which the animal's follicles are stimulated is estimated.

The nature of the feedback action of the rising levels of oestrogen on FSH production is obviously central to any analysis of the situation.

The relationship could be one of the following:

1   A negative feedback, but with a sharp 'cut-off' point rather than a continuous inhibition. On this view, FSH levels would rise unchecked until the resulting rise in oestrogens (probably oestradiol) reached the 'threshold' level for the mechanism in the pituitary (or hypothalamus above), when there would be a sharp drop in FSH and then, in turn, in oestrogen. This has been the popular view for the last fifteen years or so, although it sounds a rather unlikely physiological mechanism. However, does the recent data given in Figure 15 support this?

2   Direct control of timing from the hypothalamus. Hypothalamic 'clocks' seem to exist; this could be one. There would be no direct oestrogen feedback onto FSH secretion, the levels of the latter would be determined by a neurological mechanism in the hypothalamus.

This view is plausible, but unpopular, because it still leaves the workings of the 'clock' to be explained, and because so much endocrine control is now known to be based on feedback mechanisms.

3   A positive feedback. More FSH gives more oestrogen which gives more FSH, until something explosive such as rupture and ovulation intervenes. However, this does not fit the facts as shown in Figure 15.

Thus it is not yet possible to be sure how the rise and fall of the oestrogen levels is achieved, though it may become a little clearer as we consider the rest of the cycle. Before doing so, we should consider the effects of the rising levels of oestrogen on the rest of the system.

Moderately high and rising levels of oestrogen promote the invasion of tissue, especially reproductive tract tissue, by blood vessels. Thus throughout the first half of the cycle the vascularization of the endometrium and other tissues including the mammary glands takes place quite rapidly. It also makes the uterine muscle become rather active, contracting spontaneously from time to time, and greatly increases its sensitivity to the hormone oxytocin (Unit 9, Appendix 1).

Thus a number of the events we described in the previous Section can be accounted for by this FSH/oestrogen system. However, if an animal with the pituitary removed (an hypophysectomized animal) is given increasing FSH doses at physiological levels*, although the follicles ripen and secrete, and the genital tract proceeds to the day 15/16 appearance, ovulation does not take place. If, however, a small dose of a second pituitary gonadotrophin called luteinizing hormone (LH) is added when there are ripe follicles, even a reduced dose of FSH is sufficient to allow ovulation. LH by itself will not ripen and rupture the follicles.

LH

This is an example of an important effect quite often seen in hormone action, when two hormones combine to give an effect greater than they could produce singly—even in higher dosage. The effect is known as *synergism*.

synergism

It appears that the LH becomes in effect the 'dominant' gonadotrophin for the second part of the oestrous cycle, except in a few animals, such as the rat, which

---

* '*Physiological levels.*' *A term meaning that the amount of the substance artificially introduced results in a level of it in the blood or tissue comparable to that which could be achieved by natural means. This is in contrast to 'pharmacological levels', which implies a very much larger dose. It is a very important distinction in the interpretation of research results. For example, the natural synergism of oestrogen+progesterone on the endometrium and mammary gland can often be mimicked by the injection of oestrogen alone if it is in doses much larger than could occur naturally.*

require a third gonadotrophin (luteotrophic hormone, also called prolactin) to activate the corpus luteum. In other mammals, the LH has the effect of promoting the development of the corpus luteum from the original granulosa cells of the follicle.

prolactin

Endothelial nuclei of capillary   Nuclei of luteal cells

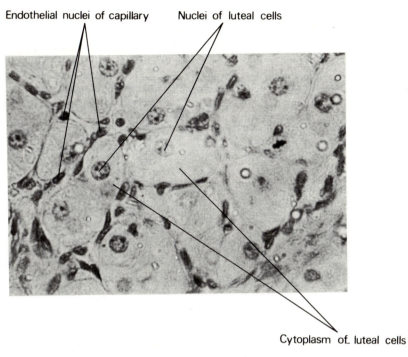

Cytoplasm of luteal cells

Figure 16   *High power photomicrograph of corpus luteum.*

Referring to Figures 4 and 16, what type of activity would you consider most likely for the corpus luteum?

Further steroid secretion, oestrogen or other.

Figure 15 suggests strongly that the function of the corpus luteum may be the secretion of a little oestradiol and a lot of progesterone, which is another steroid (see p. 16) with complex effects on the cycle. Firstly it appears to have a negative feedback relationship with LH, which results in fairly steady levels of progesterone in pregnancy, but in the normal oestrous cycle this state is not reached. It seems quite probable that other factors intervene to destroy the corpus luteum before a steady state is reached—we will consider this point again.

progesterone

The progesterone acts with the now rather lowered level of oestrogen to take the lining of the uterus to a state where it will accept the blastocyst if it arrives.

What is this type of co-ordinated effect called?

Synergism.

For the surface of the endometrium to be receptive, there must have been oestrogen 'pre-treatment', followed by just the right number of hours of oestrogen plus progesterone.*

> * *In the strain of rat with a 4-day oestrous cycle, an animal on which much of this work has been done, it has been found that a short 'burst' of oestrogen secretion, released at 18.00 hours on the 4th day after fertilization, is necessary for really satisfactory implantation. This oestrogen release, of course, follows the normal priming with oestrogen plus progesterone. Implantation will take place before this oestrogen burst, but less firmly and with a much higher failure rate. It is possible that, in this species, the oestrogen 'burst' is really associated with the ripening of the follicles of the next cycle. Thus, although it is thought that the endometrium of most mammals can be made receptive by oestrogen priming followed by oestrogen plus progesterone synergism for an appropriate period, in the rat it appears to be: oestrogen⟶oestrogen plus progesterone⟶24-hour interval⟶oestrogen, for best results. This might be a special situation in small animals, related to the shortness of the cycle compared with the time taken for the ovum to pass down the Fallopian tube, form a blastocyst and begin to implant.*

21

Most interesting, however, is the strongly *antagonistic* action of the progesterone on the oestrogen stimulation of the uterine muscle. The progesterone softens the muscle and relaxes the tone, reducing the spontaneous contractions.

antagonism

From what has been said, would you expect progesterone to act synergistically or antagonistically on the mammary glands?

Synergistically. You recall that at this stage the glands develop fast. In fact, whereas the oestrogen promoted vascular growth, oestrogen plus progesterone gives rapid growth of the milk ducts and alveoli as well.

The progesterone also appears to inhibit the development of new follicles, presumably by inhibiting FSH, though this has not been shown. However, it is quite possible that some LH is necessary in a normal animal even to produce the pre-ovulatory follicular growth and secretion of oestrogen (Fig. 15), and a high progesterone level certainly seems to inhibit LH secretion, so this may be the mechanism. (The second oestrogen peak seems to come from the corpus luteum not from new follicles.) This effect could have a considerable selective value; it is not desirable to ovulate and possibly start another pregnancy when one is under way, though this happens very occasionally.

ITQ 2 If a woman ate a mixture of oestradiol and progesterone each day of the cycle from day 3 to day 26, the dose being sufficient to maintain a blood level comparable to the peak levels shown in Figure 15, what effect do you think this would have on the ovarian cycle?

Read the answer to ITQ 2 (p. 35).

This woman is, of course, effectively on 'the pill'—though in practice the mixture would be of synthetic steroids, with greater activity, fewer side-effects—and would be cheaper.

the contraceptive pill

ITQ 3 What would you expect the overall effect on the oestrous cycle to be if this 'pill' were taken continuously, every day of every cycle?

ITQ 4 What effect might this 'pill' have on implantation, should ovulation and fertilization occur in spite of inhibition of the gonadotrophins?

Read the answers to ITQs 3 and 4 (p. 35).

ITQ 5 It is possible to take a very small dose of synthetic progesterone every day of the year, too small to interrupt the normal cycle, but apparently enough to prevent pregnancy. Can you think how this can be working?

Read the answer to ITQ 5 (p. 35).

8.3.3 The life of the corpus luteum

We have been discussing the role of progesterone, and have mentioned that the corpus luteum regresses towards the end of the cycle if implantation does not occur. This is a very fascinating and important fact, and there has been much speculation as to the cause of the breakdown of the corpus luteum (luteolysis).

Whatever the mechanism of luteolysis, the control of it to *retain* the corpus luteum in pregnancy represents, physiologically, the main difference between the placental mammals and the marsupials (the pouched mammals such as the kangaroo and the opossum (Fig. 17)). In other respects the marsupial reproductive process is similar to that of the placentals, but the 'implantation' of the blastocyst is only temporary. Pregnancy only lasts for the remainder of the cycle, though this may be a little prolonged. Then luteolysis occurs, followed by rising oestrogen and ovulation—at least in the kangaroo. The very early embryo is therefore thrust out 'willy-nilly' so to speak, and must wriggle into the pouch, where it anchors itself to the teat of the mammary gland. In the kangaroo, the embryo, only an inch or so long, wriggles along a ridge of upward pointing hairs on the mother's abdomen which run towards the pouch. The embryo can do

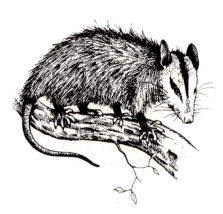

Figure 17 *Opossum.*

22

this without help from its mother partly because of the precocious development of its forelimbs—unexpected in a kangaroo! The mother licks her belly just before the birth so the young almost swims upwards to the pouch.

Clearly then there is great evolutionary significance in the change from a mechanism whereby the corpus luteum 'automatically' regresses, to one where it can remain and prolong the progestational, and perhaps gestational endometrium. Before we can appreciate this change, we must know why the corpus luteum regresses—what ends its activity?

If one favours a hypothalamic 'clock' as the determinant of the sequence of gonadotrophin secretion, then there is no conceptual difficulty—only the problem of proving it. On this theory, LH can be 'switched off' after so many days, much as it was 'switched on' to produce ovulation. (Actually 'on' and 'off' are both relative terms, as some LH secretion seems to occur throughout the oestrous cycle.) However, there are some difficulties in this hypothesis. How does implantation act so rapidly (within a few days in women) to prevent the cessation of LH release? The blastocyst is unlikely to be able to react with the endometrium as early as this, to produce a hormone which feeds back to the hypothalamus and maintains LH secretion.

hypothalamic clock

It has been shown in sheep that if the nerves leading to and from the uterus are cut, implantation does not succeed. This could possibly be a pathway, but it has not been followed up with such an interpretation in mind—as we said above, hypothalamic clocks have lacked credibility among most workers.

Most efforts have been concentrated on trying to explain the termination of the corpus luteum on a feedback basis, but it has not been easy.

One can postulate that the peak level of progesterone causes a 'cut-off', on the lines which have been suggested for oestrogen and FSH secretion just prior to ovulation, but the experimental evidence gives no support for this.

However, since it is implantation in the endometrium which leads to the prevention of luteolysis, it is not unreasonable to look at the uterus to see if it contains the normal cause of luteolysis. It was shown that surgical removal of the uterus after ovulation led to a great extension in the life of the corpora lutea.

uterus

ITQ 6　What conclusion do you draw from this experiment?

Read the answer to ITQ 6 (p. 35).

The findings are surprising in that they imply that the timing of the whole cycle is dependent on a uterine mechanism—i.e. that after a certain number of days (depending on species) of progesterone secretion, the uterus releases hormone X which stops the cycle and allows a new one to begin.

A further experiment, however, produced even more surprising results. The removal of *one* horn of a bicornuate uterus resulted in the persistence of the corpus luteum in the ovary on the side of the animal from which the horn had been removed, while on the intact side the corpora lutea regressed at the end of the cycle in the normal way.

ITQ 7　Is this compatible with the interpretation of the previous experiment?

Read the answer to ITQ 7 (p. 35).

Following the publication of these results, several workers have begun to look for a possible pathway, as well as for the substance itself. Some very interesting results are just beginning to emerge, although as yet (1972) the story is by no means fully clear.

On the anatomical side of the investigation, it has been found that branches of the uterine veins, which carry the blood draining from the uterus, do in fact run very close to the ovarian artery, shortly before it reaches the ovary. In some cases the vein actually coils around the artery. This could be a point at which substances from the uterus could diffuse into the ovarian circulation.

The chemical side of the investigation has also produced exciting results. It has been found that towards the end of the oestrous cycle, a substance known as 'prostaglandin'* can be isolated from the uterus in considerable quantities. If extracted prostaglandin is perfused into the ovarian artery, luteolysis occurs.

prostaglandin

It is quite clear that these initial results do not yet form proof of anything, and that, as so commonly is the case, they pose more questions than they answer. For example, why the destruction of the corpus luteum and not of all the steroid secretory tissue? Why should prostaglandin but not all the CO_2 and waste products cross from the vein to the artery? What times the production and release of prostaglandin from the uterus? Are other substances, such as steroids, using this pathway? (It is known that later in pregnancy the placenta is a major source of steroids.) This work has undoubtedly opened up a whole fascinating chapter in reproductive research. When first isolated, it seemed that prostaglandin worked as a purely intracellular substance, or at most a 'parahormone' by our earlier definition; it may well be, however, that we have to promote it to 'hormone' status.

8.3.4 Release of the gonadotrophins

In Section 8.3.2 we looked at the co-ordination of the oestrous cycle by the gonadotrophins, FSH and LH, from the pituitary, and also at their relationship with the steroids of the oestrogen, androgen and progesterone groups. When discussing the feedback effects of these steroids, we did not commit ourselves as to the site of action—whether it was the pituitary itself, or the hypothalamus above it.

You will recall that the pituitary also secretes other 'trophic' hormones (hormones which act on glands to stimulate the secretion of their hormones); the one you will be familiar with from S100, Unit 18 is TSH (thyroid stimulating hormone). In the case of TSH, it appears that its manufacture and release depend on the production of another chemical factor—by neurosecretory cells in the hypothalamus. This factor, which we called TRF, finds its way from the neurosecretory cells of the hypothalamus to the secretory cells of the anterior lobe of the pituitary (the part of the pituitary responsible for all the trophic hormones) in the small portal blood system which connects the two regions. If you cut through the pituitary stalk connecting the gland with the hypothalamus, and separate the two cut surfaces with a slip of waxed paper, TRF will not reach the pituitary. In this event, the release of TSH from the gland virtually ceases, and there is little or no variation in response to changes in the level of thyroxin released by the thyroid and circulating in the blood. From this we can conclude that the most important site of action of the circulating thyroxin is in the hypothalamus, not directly on the pituitary gland.

hypothalamic releasing factors

The same appears to be true of gonadotrophin release. FSH and LH release ceases if the above operation is performed, with the result that the ovaries regress and oestrogen production falls to the same very low base level reached if the whole pituitary is removed. In the course of 1971, a neurosecretory substance was isolated from the hypothalamus of pigs. This substance promoted the rapid release of both LH and FSH when injected into intact animals and into women, and in incubated isolated pituitaries. The substance has been provisionally called FSH/LH-releasing hormone (FSH/LH–RH), and it is a polypeptide (a decapeptide), the amino-acid sequence of which is known; it has been manu-

FSH/LH–RH

---

* '*Prostaglandin*' *is as yet a very enigmatic substance. It derived its name from its initial discovery in the prostate gland, but it is now known to occur in very many tissues of the body, in both sexes. Its natural functions in the body are still little understood, but concentrates of it, when injected into the blood stream, produce vigorous contractions of the uterine muscle, and are particularly effective in causing the expulsion of implanted blastocysts or even embryos at quite an advanced stage. For this reason it is being investigated as a possible major aid in the control of fertility. It appears to be harmless in the correct dosage and, if taken by mouth, might prove to be an ideal 'once a month' pill for contraceptive purposes.*

factured synthetically. At the moment, therefore, there appears to be only a single factor concerned in the release of both FSH and LH, but LH release is three times more sensitive to it than is FSH release. It may well be that whether LH or FSH release is dominant at any point depends on the circulating steroid dominant at the time—however, there is much still to be done before the picture is quite clear.

8.3.5 Control of male reproductive function

It is to be expected that there will be broad similarities between the hormonal control of reproductive function in both sexes; the sex glands arise from the same embryonic tissues, the neurosecretory centres in the brain appear to be the same, as do the structures within the pituitary. The female has circulating androgens (0.1 μg per 100 cm^3 plasma, compared to 0.5 μg in males) and the urine of normal males contains the equivalent of 50 international units of oestrone per day (compared with about 500 i.u. in a female at ovulation), so really we are probably looking at different variations of the same type of mechanism.

The male has no cycle comparable to the oestrous cycle of the female, so what has to be co-ordinated is the equivalent of maturation of the ovum, including meiosis, and ovulation, i.e. the process of ripening and shedding of sperm into the lumen of the seminiferous tubules; also the development and maintenance of the secondary sexual characters. In the case of seasonal breeders, these characters may be varied in and out of the season, and spermatogenesis will be linked to the season, just as is oogenesis and ovulation.

The male pituitary secretes both FSH and LH, but not in a monthly cycle; secretion is more or less continuous during the breeding season, which in many species may, of course, be all the year round. If the animal is hypophysectomized, the testes regress (in some species they are withdrawn into the abdominal cavity), the epithelium of the seminiferous tubules, which normally produces the sperm, breaks up and meiosis ceases; the Leydig cells between the tubules **Leydig cells** (Fig. 7, p. 14) become reduced, and the testicular androgens (for example, *testosterone*) are no longer secreted, which in many species results in the loss of the secondary sexual characteristics.

If pure FSH is administered soon after hypophysectomy in the rat, spermatogenesis is not maintained for long, and the Leydig cells decline, with loss of testosterone. However, the large *Sertoli cells* in the epithelium of the tubules, **Sertoli cells** (Fig. 6, p. 14) which are believed to nourish and sustain the developing sperm cells and spermatids until they are fully ripe, are unaffected. They remain large, active and secretory. This is rather interesting because they are derived from cells in the embryo identical to those that give rise to the follicular cells (granulosa cells) of the ovary. In the female, they sustain the ovum and, as you know, they respond to FSH; they grow and also secrete oestrogen and are generally thought to be the source of most of the ovarian oestrogen. You might think that the Sertoli cells would therefore be likely candidates as the source of testosterone, but it seems that the major source is, in fact, the Leydig cells; however, there is some testicular oestrogen—perhaps it comes from the Sertoli cells.

If pure LH is given to a recently hypophysectomized rat, spermatogenesis is **LH** maintained for a considerable period, and androgen-secretion by the Leydig cells continues for very long periods. However, for spermatogenesis to continue indefinitely, both FSH and LH must be given. The main effect of LH is due to its action in causing testosterone secretion; if you give FSH plus androgen, it is nearly as effective in maintaining a functional testis (except, of course, for the Leydig cells). In fact, androgen alone will maintain the tubules for a considerable time, but spermatogenesis eventually declines; this could be an effect involving the Sertoli cells, though some workers believe that LH is directly necessary in the long term for successful meiosis.

Thus, to summarize the evidence provided by the present work, FSH is rather limited in its action, which is confined mainly to the Sertoli cells. LH is of the greatest importance, largely as the stimulus for androgen secretion, with which it has a negative feedback relationship. It may also be important in acting directly on the germinal epithelium, possibly in some stages of meiosis.

It is likely that both androgen feedback and extrinsic factors act on LH secretion via the same or similar hypothalamic pathways as in the female, but it is not yet known whether the same FSH/LH releasing hormone is involved.

testis temperature

The glands involved in the production of the seminal fluid, including the prostate, Cowper's glands and the seminal vesicles, are dependent on adequate androgen levels and therefore on LH.

If the testes are kept at the full body temperature by insulating the scrotum or retaining the testes surgically in the abdomen, the germinal epithelium degenerates. Even in those mammals where they do not normally descend, the testes move to the outer edge of the abdominal wall where they are measurably cooler in the breeding season; they degenerate if warmed. The reason for this degeneration is not clear, and until it is we cannot even guess at what must be a fascinating evolutionary story. In mammals with a scrotum, there is a counter-current heat exchanger, the *pampiniform plexus*, involving the blood supply to the testes; it operates on the same principle as the system in a duck's leg (Unit 6, Appendix 2). The blood vessels of this plexus are selectively destroyed by the administration of cadmium salts, thus allowing the temperature of the testes to rise and the germinal epithelium to degenerate. Cadmium has therefore been under consideration as a male contraceptive but has not been used because the effect is irreversible (or may be), there are possible side effects and also because vasectomy (cutting the vas deferens) seems simpler and safer.

cadmium salts

8.3.6 Summary of Section 8.3

In this Section we first described the steroid nucleus—the 'body' of the steroid hormones, and very briefly made a number of important generalizations about steroid hormones, including: the chemical similarity of physiologically dissimilar hormones, the fact that one hormone may be the precursor of another, the distinction between steroids produced and secreted as part of a physiological response and those which were breakdown products excreted in the urine or man-made synthetics.

In the bulk of the Section we considered the hormonal regulation of the mammalian female cycle; the parts played by steroids in changes in the reproductive tract; the relationship of the steroids to the gonadotrophins which control their release; the factors responsible for gonadotrophin release, though not the regulation of the factors.

The general conclusions were that FSH, probably in conjunction with a fairly low level of LH (synergistic action), was responsible for follicular growth (FSH) and oestrogen secretion (FSH and LH). The oestrogen thus released produced changes in the reproductive tract, mammary glands and behaviour, though the last point was not stressed. A sharp LH peak was required to produce ovulation, and continued LH (in the rat, prolactin) was needed to cause progesterone production by the corpus luteum. The LH/progesterone system inhibited the ripening of further follicles, but some oestrogen is produced towards the latter part of the cycle. It is the sharp fall in the steroid levels, particularly the oestrogens, which causes the shedding of the endometrium, as visible menstruation in females of the higher primates. The factors affecting the life of the corpus luteum, and thus the duration of the cycle, in pregnant and non-pregnant animals were considered on the basis of:

1 a hypothalamic 'clock';
2 'conventional' views of steroid feedback;
3 recent evidence of 'local factors'.

In male mammals, spermatogenesis and the development of secondary sexual characters are under hormonal control. FSH affects Sertoli cells that nourish developing sperm. LH stimulates androgen-production by Leydig cells and there is a feedback mechanism probably via thalamic pathways similar to those of the female. Androgens control secondary sexual characters. Spermatogenesis is very sensitive to temperature.

26

8.4 Effects of Extrinsic Factors on the Hormonal Regulation of the Cycle

Study Comment

Here the ways in which female mammal reproductive cycles are affected by certain events outside the animal are discussed. If you are short of time you should read through this Section quickly.

8.4.1 Induced ovulation

We have been considering some of the ways in which reproductive hormones may act and interact, but only on a purely internal basis—all the factors involved being within the body. Any system of co-ordination will serve the organism much better if it not only regulates physiological activities in relation to internal factors, but also co-ordinates them with environmental factors. One environmental (or anyway, extrinsic) factor of consequence to the efficacy of the female reproductive system is the supply of fresh sperm; it is of obvious advantage if the hormonally-controlled cycle is integrated with the arrival of sperm in the tract, or failing that, at least with the appearance of a suitable male. There is some evidence of integration in the latter case, which we mention briefly below when dealing with pheromones. With regard to the former case, a number of mammals do in fact co-ordinate ovulation with mating. These include cats, rabbits and ferrets, and they are called induced ovulators. The animals stay in a state of almost permanent oestrous throughout their breeding season which, for example, in the ferret is from spring until early September or thereabouts (in the domesticated strains of these animals various changes may occur—oestrous may be almost permanent, as in the domestic rabbit, or intermittent). Then ten hours after mating, ovulation occurs.

induced ovulators

In rabbits, ovulation does *not* occur after mating if any of the following procedures are adopted prior to mating:

1 The sensory nerves from the cervix and nearby pelvic areas are cut.

2 Local anaesthetic is applied to the cervix and genital areas.

3 Drugs which block the transmission of nerve impulses from one nerve to another (e.g. atropine, dibenamine) are injected into the hypothalamus (in this case, up to one minute after mating).

4 The pituitary stalk is cut and waxed paper inserted.

5 The pituitary is removed.

If, on the other hand, one or several of the procedures 1–4 is adopted, but not until ten minutes or so after mating, ovulation will still occur ten hours later. Procedure 5 may in some cases prevent ovulation if carried out within half an hour of mating.

> **ITQ 8** What do you think the mechanism is that causes ovulation, having regard to the above data?

Read the answer to ITQ 8 (p. 35).

Evidence from other mammals would lead one to expect that the pituitary hormone involved in this case would be LH. This does indeed prove to be the case. As the above experiments showed, the initial release of LH is very quick, and the duration of LH secretion need not be long; however, the necessary changes in the wall of the ripe follicle seem to take longer (10 hours) whether there is only a short 'burst' of LH or a longer one.

LH

> **ITQ 9** Can you think why induced ovulation might offer a selective advantage over the 'normal' mechanism?

Read the answer to ITQ 9 (p. 35).

The 'normal' system, whereby ovulation occurs at a particular point of the oestrous cycle regardless of mating, is called *spontaneous ovulation*. This may be a very misleading phrase. The pathways involved in spontaneous ovulation are similar to the ones described above, except for the part played by the sensory nerves from the pelvis. The hypothalamus is involved in the timing of the release

spontaneous ovulation

of LH/FSH releasing hormone, and thus of LH itself. In rats, which are spontaneous ovulators, there is a sensory component from the cervix involved in keeping the corpus luteum secreting progesterone, though not in ovulation itself. A single female rat will usually ovulate normally, complete the cycle and enter oestrous again. If after ovulation you stimulate the cervix with a glass rod, the corpus luteum is retained and pseudopregnancy follows.

It is almost certain that there is a hypothalamic clock timing ovulation in rats. Those with a 5-day oestrous cycle ovulate between 1 and 2 o'clock in the morning of the fourth day. LH release occurs between 2 pm and 4 pm the previous day. If the animal is lightly anaesthetized with phenobarbitone between 2 and 4 pm on the day before ovulation, ovulation does not occur—and if this is repeated between 2 and 4 pm each subsequent day, ovulation does not occur at all. On the other hand, this clock can be made to run 'fast' by 24 hours if the steroid levels are appropriately raised on the second or third day. The fact that even in a spontaneous ovulator, there is a delicate hypothalamic timing device means that potentially ovulation is open to influence by a number of extrinsic factors, if they affect the hypothalamus. Clearly however this clock is influenced by the steroid levels in the blood.

hypothalamic clock

8.4.2   Light and temperature

As we said earlier in this Unit, many animals come into oestrous only at certain times of year, and the males of the species only develop active testes at this period. The biological significance is obvious, and has already been mentioned. What regulates this periodicity?

From what you know already, you would expect that the animal will begin to come into season as a result of rising levels of FSH/LH in the blood. This will cause follicular growth and oestrogen secretion, resulting in secondary sexual factors such as enlargements of the genetalia, sexual behaviour, mating plumage in birds, etc. The question then really is, what starts FSH/LH secretion? Again you know the answer—neurosecretion and the production of FSH/LH releasing hormone by cells in the hypothalamus. What causes this? A large number of nerve tracts enter the hypothalamus, so it could be many nervous factors, or it could be an 'annual clock' or it could be a chemical in the blood.

The evidence is that in most seasonally breeding vertebrates the onset of the breeding cycle is connected with day-length or average temperature or, frequently, with both. Even in the rat, which is thought of as an animal which cycles continuously, an increased period of daylight will prolong oestrous, and continuous dark from birth will delay sexual maturity, and may cause periods of anoestrous.

day-length

In sheep, as with many animals, it is not the absolute length of the day which is material but *changes* in day-length. Thus as the days shorten by a certain amount each 24 hours, the animals begin to secrete FSH and LH (Fig. 18).

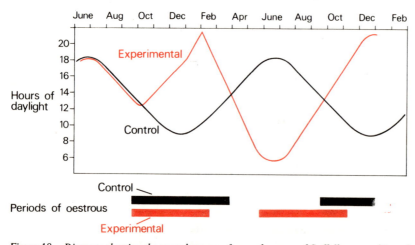

Figure 18   *Diagram showing the sexual season of several groups of Suffolk ewes subjected to different lighting conditions. The sexual season in each case is shown as a solid band beneath the corresponding light curve. In all cases oestrus started 10–14 weeks after the change-over from increasing to decreasing light.*

The same is true of deer—another species of 'short day breeder'—but many mammals, such as the horse, come into season with the lengthening days and are sometimes called 'long day breeders'. Many birds are sensitive in the same way, and the weight of the gonads (which regress out of season) and plumage changes can be used to measure the onset of gonadotrophin secretion. In Britain, most birds are long day breeders. Other factors such as food supply may be very important in birds.

It seemed reasonable to investigate the possibility that the eyes were the main receptors, and in many animals this has proved to be the case; there are receptors in the retina, and if the optic nerve is cut, or the eyes covered, the response is abolished. Exactly how the amount of stimulation received by these receptors is compared over a period of days and weeks is not yet known. Clearly an element of neurological 'memory' enters into it.

However, the receptors are not always in the eyes. In some ducks the receptors have been shown to occur in the skin around the eyes. In some birds, response to the photoperiod (day-length) continued even though all the sensory pathways from the eyes and surface of the head were blocked. Remarkable though it seems, it appeared that light was reaching the hypothalamus directly, through the feathers and skull. Photosensitive measuring devices implanted in the hypothalamus confirmed this; apparently the light can be converted into an interpretable signal inside the brain as well as in the retina.

In the same way, it has been shown that sunlight can reach the hypothalamus of sheep, though exactly what effect this has is uncertain. If continuous light is conducted into the hypothalamus of a blinded rat down 'optical fibres', it will enter an extended oestrous just as will a rat given the same light treatment with its eyes intact. A blinded rat without the 'optical fibres' tends to go into anoestrous, or cycle more or less normally.

The pineal gland, in mammals a vestige of the 'pineal eye' still visible in the tuatara (*Sphenodon*) a primitive reptile (*S100*, Units 19 and 21), is important in this respect. Some mammals, for example the ferret, will go into almost permanent oestrous regardless of the day-length if the pineal is removed. It may be that changes in day-length affect inhibition of the gonadotrophins by pineal hormones.

8.4.3 Delayed implantation

The effects of varying day-length may do more than simply bring animals into season, or out of it. In some cases, the fertilized blastocysts do not implant but remain free in the uterus until changes in the day-length occur; then implantation occurs normally. In this way, animals of some species mate in the spring, delay implantation until autumn or winter, and give birth the following spring. Alternatively, those with shorter gestation periods (e.g. the hedgehog) mate in the late summer and delay implantation with the result that the young are born in the early spring. The roe deer and the European badger can delay implantation for more than four months, and this delay can be terminated by changing the photoperiod. The exact mechanism is unknown, and it is difficult to reproduce experimentally.

In rats which have had their ovaries removed immediately after ovulation and mating, the fertilized blastocysts will stay alive but free for up to two months if the animal is given a continuous, low dose of progesterone. If this is then supplemented with more progesterone and oestrogen, implantation often occurs. However, this may not mirror the steroid pattern in animals which naturally show delayed implantation.

In the kangaroo—a marsupial—the young are born at the end of the oestrous cycle. They transfer to the pouch, and attach themselves to the teat. The mother immediately cycles again and mates—this is called post-partum mating. The fertilized blastocyst does not implant, but survives for several months. If during that time the baby in the pouch dies, or is taken off the teat permanently, the blastocyst implants and develops. The hormonal background is not clear, nor whether suckling is producing changes in the pattern of secretion similar to those produced by day-length in other animals.

Women are rather infertile while suckling babies. This has been assumed to be due to reduced ovulation; it would be interesting to see if it were really due to less successful implantation.

8.4.4 Pheromones

As we said at the beginning of the Unit, pheromones are substances released into the environment that affect other individuals which pick them up. They are usually airborne, and are therefore said to be smelled. So far as mammals are concerned, there are functionally two different types, those which affect the nervous system only, and thus short-term behaviour, and those which affect the endocrine balance, perhaps with rather longer-term effects. This distinction may be arbitrary; too little is known about the mechanism of either response to make a very meaningful classification. We deal with those affecting mating behaviour very briefly in the TV programme of this Unit. Remember that the sex hormones also control the secretion of these pheromones.

With regard to the effects of pheromones on the reproductive cycle, some of the earliest observations were made on mice. It was shown that caging females together in small groups could lead to pseudopregnancies, and in large groups to periods of anoestrous. A group of females will synchronize their cycles if a male of the same strain is introduced into the cage.

mice

If a male of a strange strain is introduced into a cage with females which have been recently mated, the blastocysts do not implant successfully, and the number of pregnancies is drastically reduced. It can be shown that the normal oestrogen/progesterone pattern is disrupted, so the effect is clearly via the gonadotrophin-releasing hormone and the gonadotrophins. If the olfactory nerve is cut in the females prior to the introduction of the male, normal pregnancies are achieved. The biological value to the species of this mechanism is not immediately apparent.

8.4.5 Summary of Section 8.4

To summarize this Section, it is clear that a number of external stimuli can have an effect on the reproductive hormones, and that this effect is to relate events in the cycle to events outside the animal. In all the mechanisms so far studied, the external stimulus has acted via the neurosecretory system in the hypothalamus. This appears also to be the case where diet and temperature are major factors—it is noteworthy that the temperature-regulating centre and the 'hunger' and 'satiety' centres are located in the hypothalamus, and direct nervous connections could easily exist between them and the neurosecretory cells.

A summary of the relationship between the hypothalamus and the gonads is given in Figure 19.

8.5 The Determination of Sex and Sexual Characters

Study Comment

This short Section concerns the relationship between genetic sex and hormones. It illustrates a 'one-off' effect of reproductive hormones. You could omit this if short of time.

Some very interesting examples of 'once for all' actions of hormones are to be found in the determination of sexual characters.

On casual consideration it is easy to assume that the definitive sex of a phenotype is determined by its genotype, and that the appropriate sex hormones, themselves determined by the genotype, merely produce the more superficial secondary sexual characteristics. Such an assumption would, however, be a gross oversimplification.

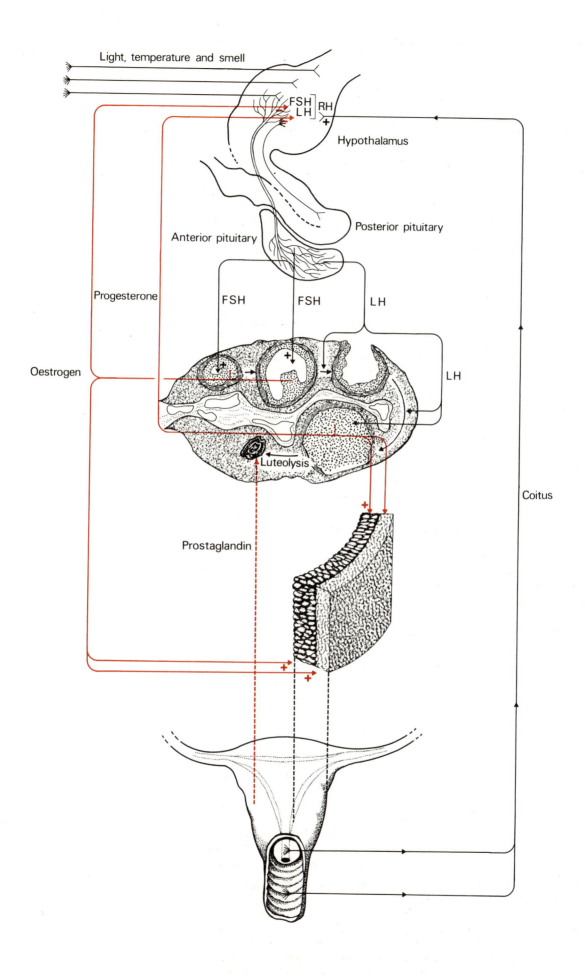

Figure 19   *Diagrammatic summary of gonadotrophins and steroid target organs.*

There are various systems of genotypic sex determination: mammals, many frogs, some teleost fishes and dipterous insects (the two-winged flies) show what you may think of as the 'normal' system, the female being homozygous for the sex chromosomes (XX) and the male heterozygous (XY). However, birds show the reverse situation, the male being ZZ and the female ZW (these are sometimes referred to as XX and XY also, but the above notation avoids confusion), as do reptiles, some amphibians, some fishes and many insects. In some species there may be an XX (female) and XO (male). It is known that in *Drosophila* 'super females' may occur (XXY), but in human beings, XXY gives a phenotypic male.

It can be shown experimentally that in teleost fish, the 'genetic sex' may be completely overriden by appropriate hormone treatment. The medaka (*Oryzias latipes*) has the 'mammal' system XX (♀) and XY (♂). It is viviparous, and if the young males are treated with oestrogens they develop into fully functional females, with all the sexual apparatus. Such XY 'females' can be bred normally with XY males, giving some YY offspring. These, of course, give all male (XY) offspring when mated with normal females (XX). The identical but opposite procedure may also be performed using androgens giving fully functional males with XX chromosomes, which when mated with normal females give only XX offspring. Thus if the treatment is given at the right time, the genetic sex is irrelevant—fully functional gonads of the 'wrong' kind can be induced, and they will produce the 'wrong' gametes and 'wrong' sex hormones.

Complete reversal can also be obtained in the African clawed toad (*Xenopus*), turning genetic males into fully functional females by oestrogen treatment at a critical period.

Mammals can be induced to produce testes in a genetic female or ovaries in a genetic male, but so far experiments of this kind have not produced total, functional reversal of the anatomy, possibly because more of the genital anatomy is genetically determined. 'Free-martins' are a case in point. Free-martins are sterile female calves, with normal female external genitalia but testes and male ducts internally. A free-martin is produced only if her placenta establishes a cross-circulation with the placenta of a male twin calf while in the uterus of the mother.

They are rare because (a) twinning is uncommon in cows; (b) if both twins are female, both are normal; (c) sometimes even if the twin is male, the placentas do not overlap. It seems that androgenic substances from the bull-calf affect the ovaries, turning them into testes, but that the female external genitalia remains. (The genitalia remain immature in the adult free-martin, owing to lack of oestrogen.) What then normally determines whether an ovary or a testes will develop in the appropriate genetic sex?

It seems established that in the embryo of either genetic sex the primordial germ cells can develop into ova or sperm. These primordial cells move by amoeboid action into an area called the genital ridge, which later forms the gonad. The primordial cells which develop in the outer cortex of this ridge form ova, those in the inner medulla form sperm. Normally of course, *either* the medulla *or* the cortex, with their complement of germ cells, will develop, but not both. Whichever one develops will suppress the other.

While this information leads us close to the point at which genetic sex must be determining phenotypic sex, it leaves us still just too far away. Some workers believe that they have shown that the cortex of the ridge produces one parahormone and the medulla another. The hormone produced is determined by the genetic sex, and the part which produces it 'wins'; the primordial germ cells which have entered it become the appropriate gametes. It is certainly true that if you take two embryos of opposite genetic sexes, and remove the primordial germ cells from one and plant them in the gential ridge of the other, they will functionally adopt the sex of the latter. Thus the primordial germ cells from the genetic female will end up as sperm, as in the androgen-treated fish and frogs.

It seems fairly certain therefore that under natural circumstances, hormones determine the sex of all the reproductive system in lower vertebrates, and of the gonads themselves in mammals, though the external genitalia may be genetically determined in the latter. Normally, of course, the genetic sex determines which hormones will be produced in the embryo, so the two effects go hand in hand. Not all of the 'determining' effects of sex hormones are this difficult to assess. In the case of some of the secondary sexual characters it is quite a simple matter to compare the effects of sex steroids with effects of differential growth determined by genotype. You may care to analyse the following observations.

1 In a breed of sheep where only the rams have horns, removal of the testes in the young ram prevents the growth of the horns. After removal of the ovaries, the young ewe does not grow horns.

2 In a breed of sheep where both sexes have horns, removal of the testes leads to the growth of the lighter 'female' type of horn, and removal of the ovaries of the ewe still leads to growth of the 'female' type of horn.

Summary of Unit 8

Here we define hormones using a modified version of the traditional definition.

They can be classified in various ways (8.1). Our treatment in Units 8, 9 and 10 is designed to illustrate four broad types of integrative action, listed in 8.1. In Unit 8, mammalian reproductive organs and cycles are described in 8.2, co-ordination of reproductive cycles in 8.3 and integration of these cycles with the outside environment in 8.4. In 8.5, a 'one-off' situation is considered.

Changes in the female reproductive tract result from the activity of steroid hormones which in turn are regulated by gonadotrophins secreted by the anterior pituitary under the control of hypothalamic 'releasing factors' (8.3). Interaction between FSH and LH is an example of synergism. The duration of the life of the corpus luteum is of paramount importance in relation to the duration of the oestrous cycle; possible control mechanisms are discussed. Male reproductive changes are associated with similar hormonal mechanisms but do not follow short period cycles.

Female reproductive cycles may be influenced by mating, by light and temperature and by pheromones (8.4).

In vertebrates, sex is basically determined by chromosomes but can be affected by hormones (8.5).

Self-assessment questions

SAQ 1 (Section 8.3.2) What effect would you expect from the continuous administration of progesterone to a female primate for at least 90 days, if the dosage were such that the level in the blood was at least that normally found on day 25 of the cycle (see Fig. 15)?

Consider the effects on: (a) the ovaries; (b) the endometrium; (c) fertility and (d) the blood levels of the naturally-secreted steroids.

SAQ 2 (Section 8.3.2) Consider the same questions as in *SAQ 1*, but assume this time that the dose of progesterone is a very low one, perhaps not more than one-tenth of that suggested in *SAQ 1*.

SAQ 3 (Sections 8.3.2 and 8.4.1) If you hypophysectomize a mature doe rabbit and soon afterwards put her in a cage with a buck, what would you have to do to make fertilization possible? If you did exactly the same experiment, but using mature rats instead of rabbits, would the same action allow fertilization to occur?

SAQ 4 (Section 8.4.1) What sort of investigations would you perform to determine whether an animal was an 'induced' or a 'spontaneous' ovulator? Is an 'induced ovulator' affected by extrinsic environmental factors so far as the cycle of events in its ovary is concerned?

SAQ 5 (Sections 8.3.2 and 8.3.5) Give two examples of the synergistic action of hormones, and one of the antagonistic action. Can the same two hormones act synergistically on one organ and antagonistically on another?

SAQ 6 (Sections 8.3.2, 8.3.4, 8.3.5 and 8.4) From what we have said in this Unit, do you feel that FSH and LH should be regarded as quite separate hormones in terms of their secretion and physiological effects?

SAQ 7 (Section 8.3.5) If you hypophysectomized a male rabbit, which of the following would you need to inject to maintain the entire reproductive system in a fully functional condition for (a) two or three weeks and (b) indefinitely?

1 FSH.   3 Progesterone.
2 LH.   4 Testosterone.

Make the assumptions that you start the injections directly after the hypophysectomy and that other pituitary factors, such as those affecting metabolism, are irrelevant.

SAQ 8 (Section 8.4.4) It has been known to farmers for many years that, in some cases, ewes may be brought into oestrous rather earlier than otherwise, by penning them next to a ram. This also has the effect of tending to synchronize their cycles to some degree. Can you think of a plausible explanation for this phenomenon?

Self-assessment Answers and Comments

SAQ 1 This is the dosage corresponding to that shown in Figure 15 as being the peak level of naturally-circulating progesterone.

You would therefore expect that (a) it would inhibit LH secretion by the pituitary and thus prevent ovulation occurring, and the lack of LH might also reduce the effect of FSH on the ripening follicles (see (d) below).

The effect (b) on the endometrium will be to maintain it in a 'progestational' state, as it will have been oestrogen-primed (and there is likely still to be some natural oestrogen in the circulation). There will be no menstruation.

The effect (c) on fertility will be to reduce it to almost nil—no ovulation and no receptive period of the endometrium.

The effects (d) on the circulating steroids may be interesting. There will be the artificially-administered progesterone, but because of its inhibitory effect on LH secretion and thus corpus luteum formation, there will be no natural luteal progesterone. As, to some extent, LH may synergize the action of FSH in causing the follicle cells to secrete increasing amounts of oestrogen, there may be a drop in the oestrogen in the blood. This effect is not visible in the short term, e.g. during the latter part of the normal cycle, but it may be one of the reasons why it has been found helpful to include oestrogen in the contraceptive 'pill'.

SAQ 2 (a) no effect.

(b) no effect on the cycle of renewal followed by shedding, and no noticeable histological changes, but see (c).

(c) fertility reduced to almost nil, apparently due to the failure of the blastocysts to implant. Thus there must, presumably, be interference with the changes to the surface of the endometrium which normally result in its 'receptive period'.

(d) no obvious effect. The administered progesterone may replace a small part of the naturally-occurring steroid by very slightly reducing the LH output, but this has not been measured.

When answering both this and the previous question, you should realize that in asking you to make firm predictions on the basis of the information in the Unit we are not saying that your answers are necessarily what happens in nature. For one thing, as you will be aware, we are working with hypotheses that have not been exhaustively tested, and by the time you read this, new information may be in the hands of the research community. For another, some of the predictions you are asked to make have not yet been fully tested, or tested only in one species. Thus in a couple of years you may find that you (and we) made the wrong prediction.

SAQ 3 Inject LH to produce ovulation. You might be able to use a smaller dose if you used an FSH/LH mixture. As the rabbit is an induced ovulator, she cannot have ovulated before hypophysectomy. In the case of the rat it will depend entirely on the stage of the oestrous cycle. If she is in oestrus, with ripe follicles, then LH injection will have the same effect as in the rabbit. If she had just ovulated anyway, nothing would be necessary to allow fertilization. If she is in some other stage of the cycle, then just an injection of LH, or even an FSH/LH mixture is most unlikely to be any use.

SAQ 4 Examine the blood or urine for signs of cyclical steroid changes; see whether fertility is affected by anaesthesia of the genitalia and cervix or by cutting the sensory nerves from the pelvic region prior to mating.

The ovary of an induced ovulator is affected by two separate classes of environmental effect—the stimulation from the male which induces the LH release for ovulation, and the normal influences of light and temperature, acting via the pituitary, which affect spontaneous and induced ovulators alike.

SAQ 5 Two examples of synergism are: (1) the effect of FSH + LH in producing ovulation (the follicle must be FSH-primed for LH to produce ovulation); (2) the action of oestrogen + progesterone on the endometrium.

Examples of antagonism are seen in the effects of oestrogens and androgens on the development of some secondary sexual characteristics.

The same hormones can display synergistic and antagonistic actions, e.g. oestrogen causes increase in the muscle tone of the uterus, with resultant spontaneous contractions, whereas progesterone causes relaxation of the muscle, enabling it to be passively stretched without reacting and largely abolishing spontaneous contractions. The two act synergistically on the endometrium.

SAQ 6 This is a difficult question. FSH and LH are distinct chemically; there appear to be differences in their feedback relationship with the levels of different steroids, and the initially higher level of FSH appears to be responsible for early follicle development, in which LH may play little part. Also there are well-established experiments indicating that FSH alone will ripen follicles, but that LH must be present for ovulation to occur. On the other hand, recent work tends to confirm the view that most of their actions are achieved synergistically, and that they are usually both present in the blood, though sometimes in rather different proportions. They also seem to share a common releasing hormone from the hypothalamus (FSH/LH releasing hormone). In the last year (1971) it has been claimed that FSH alone will cause ovulation, but this may not be in physiological doses.

On balance, the present evidence supports the view that they are functionally separate hormones, but this view is under some attack.

SAQ 7 (a) Testosterone alone will probably suffice to maintain the seminiferous tubules, spermatogenesis, and the other glands and ducts for this period. LH might be safer, as it may act directly on meiosis as well as causing testosterone release.

(b) FSH is needed for the Sertoli cells, and once again, in the long term, it is probably better to give LH than testosterone.

SAQ 8 It could be a pheromone, acting through the olfactory system and the hypothalamus to advance the cycles of those ewes not yet in oestrous. It could be a visual stimulus, but such a pathway has not yet been shown.

Answers to In-text Questions

ITQ 1 (a) Maternal blood pressure may be too high.

(b) Many immunological problems. The mother and embryo are not genetically identical, and therefore their proteins are different. The mother would develop antibodies against the embryo as if it were an invading organism.

ITQ 2 Much of the ovarian cycle will be inhibited. The continuously high level of oestradiol may well inhibit FSH secretion, if there is a negative feedback with a 'cut off' level—though we have seen that this is not certain. However, the progesterone will inhibit LH, so that even if there is enough FSH to ripen the follicles, there will be no peak of LH to cause ovulation. Also the ovarian secretion of oestrogen will be largely inhibited.

ITQ 3 The effect on the ovary will be exactly the same, but the continuously high oestrogen and progesterone will maintain the endometrium permanently in a highly developed state—more or less a 'pregnant' one. There will be no menstruation, though in practice it is found by women who do take the 'pill' continuously that there is often 'breakthrough' bleeding every three or four months. However, responses to the different synthetic steroids are individually variable.

ITQ 4 Implantation would not take place. The endometrium is only receptive for a short period if primed with oestrogen and then treated for a few hours with progesterone. This pill will produce a so-called 'progestational' uterus—comparable to that at the end of the cycle or in pregnancy—which is not receptive. This is an important point in relation to the working of the contraceptive 'pill'. It has been shown that even when it is taken regularly, occasional ovulations occur. The fact that if taken properly the failure rate is well under 1 per cent is undoubtedly due to the failure of these occasional ova to implant.

ITQ 5 This is what has been called the 'mini-pill', which has a failure rate a little higher than the conventional one. It appears that even a dose too small to interfere with LH production and the cycle will prevent the endometrium becoming receptive and implantation taking place.

The exact reason is not known but one can make suggestions. For example, the progesterone could act synergistically with the rising levels of natural oestradiol to make the receptive period come before ovulation—or perhaps *any* progesterone, too early on, results in there being *no* receptive period.

ITQ 6 A hormone or other substance is normally released by some part of the uterus, and is carried in the blood to the hypothalamus or pituitary, where it inhibits LH secretion.

Alternatively, nervous discharge occurs up the uterine nerves which inhibit LH secretion via the hypothalamus. If the latter alternative were true, however, it is suprising that cutting the nerves caused the failure of implantation in sheep (p. 23).

ITQ 7 No. Rather surprisingly, the only possible interpretation would seem to involve a *local* effect. It would appear that some substance is released from the tissue of the uterus, which finds its way *directly* to the corpus luteum. This in turn implies something comparable to a portal system, draining blood from the uterus and then carrying it to the ovary and distributing it via ovarian capillaries. No such system has been described however.

ITQ 8 A neuro-endocrine reflex. The afferent pathway would appear to be: sense organs in the genitalia and cervix (shown by procedures 1 and 2); sensory nerves (1); hypothalamus (3, also 4); neurosecretion of a releasing hormone (4); release of a pituitary hormone (5).

ITQ 9 It means that, at every mating, sperm and ova are likely to meet—whereas, in the 'normal' mechanism, many matings will be too early or too late for fertilization of the ova. It is an essentially 'economical' process.

Acknowledgements

Grateful acknowledgement is made to the following for material used in this unit:

Cambridge University Press for Figure 18 adapted from N. T. M. Yeates, *Journal of Agricultural Science*, Vol 39, No 1, 1949.

Hormones and Homeostasis:
Blood Calcium and Blood Sugar
Unit 9

Contents

Table A

List of Scientific Terms, Concepts and Principles used in Unit 9

Taken as prerequisites			Introduced in this Unit			
1 **Assumed from general knowledge**	**2** **Introduced in previous Unit**	**Unit No.**	**3** **Developed in this Unit or in its set book(s)**	**Page No.**	**4** **Developed in a later Unit**	**Unit No.**
bone	glucose	**S100** 10, 15, 16	hydroxyapatite	3		
			hypocalcaemia	3		
mammary gland	neuron	15	blood calcium	4		
	monosaccharide	15, 16	parathyroid gland	4		
	phosphorylase	15, 16	parathyroid hormone (PTH)	4		
	adrenalin	18	osteoblasts	5		
	thyroid gland	18	osteoclasts	5		
	thyroxin	18	exchangeable and non-exchangeable bone	5		
		S22	vitamin D (calciferol)	6		
	fatty acids	4	rickets	6		
	prolactin	8	calcitonin	7		
			blood sugar	8		
			hypoglycaemia	8		
			hyperglycaemia	8		
			renal threshold	8		
			insulin	9		
			islets of Langerhans	11		
			α and β cells	12		
			glucagon	12		
			lactose	19		
			adrenal cortex	19		
			glucocorticoids	20		
			mineralocorticoids	20		
			hydrocortisone	20		
			aldosterone	20		
			ACTH	21		
			adenyl cyclase	23		
			second messenger hypothesis	23		
			protein kinase	23		
			phosphorylase kinase	23		
			phosphodiesterase	25		
			colostrum	27		
			posterior pituitary	28		
			myoepithelium	28		
			oxytocin	28		

Study Guide

This is a fairly short Unit, with no set reading. Thus there is no Section that we can safely recommend you to skip, if you are short of time, except perhaps the Appendix on Lactation.

The Objectives for Unit 9 are included with those for Unit 8, with which this Unit forms a pair.

9.0 Introduction

In Unit 8, we looked at the interrelation of various hormones, with one another and with the nervous system, in the production of a complex and changing sequence of events—the reproductive cycle. We also considered examples of the maintenance of differential growth and activity by some parts of the body as a result of the continuing secretion of a hormone—for example, many of the secondary sexual characters which are sustained for as long as the relevant steroid secretion is maintained. In addition to these examples, we have seen that sometimes the action may be permanent if the hormonal secretion takes place at a critical stage of development, even if the secretion is only of short duration —as with the interaction of sex steroids with the genetic factors determining some aspects of reproductive anatomy.

An aspect of hormonal action, and a common one at that, which we have not yet considered in detail, is the effect of hormonal secretion in producing homeostatic responses. Internal homeostasis is one of the major themes of physiology; the cells of an organism must live in an environment which is regulated within narrow limits, and if the external environment in which the organism is living does not happen to fall within these limits, then internal adjustments must be made to the body fluids bathing the cells. Many factors may act to shift the composition of the body fluids beyond these limits, and substances may be constantly diffusing in or out from the environment; products of the cell's own metabolism will tend to accumulate around them; the cells will withdraw food and oxygen from the fluids.

There are many instances where hormones play a crucial part in homeostatic mechanisms; we have selected two such mechanisms for study in this Unit. We look first, rather briefly, at the way in which the calcium level of the blood is maintained within limits that allow the organism to function normally, in the face of the sometimes conflicting demands of different tissues. We then move on to look at the ways in which hormones regulate the level of blood sugar. This must be maintained within close limits, at least in mammals, if the central nervous system is to function. However, glucose and other sugars may be added to or removed from the blood very rapidly, for a variety of reasons; this calls for a very complicated and sensitive regulatory mechanism, involving nervous and hormonal integration, some aspects of which we consider in detail.

Finally in Section 9.3 we discuss something of what is known of the mode of action of the hormones on the enzyme systems within the cells they affect.

9.1 The Regulation of Calcium in the Blood Plasma

Study Comment

This Section describes the mechanism responsible for the maintenance of blood calcium. Control is effected by at least two hormones, parathyroid hormone (PTH) and calcitonin (CT). These two hormones are thought to be responsible for a type of homeostasis called a 'push-pull' mechanism.

9.1.1 The role of calcium (and phosphate) in metabolism

The absence of calcium from the diet gives rise to several metabolic disorders which give a clue to its normal cellular role. In calcium lack, or *hypocalcaemia* muscle cells respond to stimuli more readily than normal and nerve cells fire spontaneously. Powerful spontaneous or induced muscle contractions occur—a state referred to as tetany. So calcium is normally involved in the control of cell irritability, largely through its influences on the permeability of neuronal and muscle cell membranes. Calcium has other important cellular roles. It is essential for the full activity of some metabolic enzymes and it plays a key role in blood coagulation. An adequate supply of calcium is also necessary for bone formation.

hypocalcaemia

tetany

Bone is made up of mineral crystals bound together with a protein matrix. These crystals are of a substance called *hydroxyapatite* which has the formula $Ca_{10}(PO_4)_6$. Teeth are also made up of calcium and phosphate, though crystallized

3

in a rather different form, so the total body reserves of calcium and phosphate are very large indeed compared with the amount circulating in the blood. A proportion of the mineral content of the bone is in equilibrium with the calcium phosphate of the blood so blood can be thought of as being a saturated solution, so far as calcium ions (Ca_4^+) and phosphate ions ($PO_4^{\equiv}$) are concerned. This means that the addition or subtraction of one of these will affect the level of the other—if you add more PO_4 you will force some calcium out of solution. Thus we can say that the concentration of calcium in the blood is inversely related to the concentration of phosphate, or $[Ca] \times [PO_4] = K$.

Ca, Po$_4$ equlibrium

The metabolism of phosphate is intimately bound up with that of calcium. The phosphate ion has several important metabolic roles: it is an important constituent of bone; it is a component of nucleotides (which make up an important part of nucleic acids, see *S100**, Unit 17) and it is involved in the structure of membranes.

9.1.2 Calcium in the blood

Calcium occurs in blood plasma at a concentration of about 10 mg per 100 ml (10 mg%). About half of this is in a free, ionized and chemically active state. The remainder is non-ionized and bound, mainly to plasma proteins.

If calcium is injected into the mammalian blood stream, the plasma calcium concentration obviously soon rises to abnormally high values. But within about an hour, plasma calcium levels return to normal, about 10 mg%. Similarly, if calcium ions are removed from circulating blood plasma, the calcium concentration subsequently returns to normal, pre-experimental values. Blood calcium levels are regulated so finely that concentrations very rarely change by more than 5 per cent above or below normal values.

9.1.3 Parathyroid hormone

The human parathyroid glands are small yellowish oval bodies, about 6 mm long, embedded in the surface of the thyroid gland. They are very variable in size, position and number. Usually there are two pairs, but accessory parathyroid tissue is not uncommon lower in the neck, or indeed in the thorax. The vascular supply to the glands is rich, but nervous supply is scanty, transplanted parathyroid glands function normally in the absence of all nervous connection.

Following the surgical removal of mammalian parathyroid glands there is a marked fall in plasma calcium levels, and a consequent tetany. The concentration of phosphate in the plasma increases.

parathyroidectomy

The effect of an injection of a purified extract of parathyroid gland is illustrated in Figure 1a. Notice the marked rise of blood calcium and the fall in plasma phosphate. The maximum effect of the extract on phosphate concentration is reached two or three hours after injection; the maximum effect on calcium levels occurs somewhat later, about five hours after injection. The agent responsible for these changes has been extracted, purified and analysed—it is *parathyroid hormone (PTH)*.

PTH

PTH thus raises blood calcium. How is this effect achieved? Figure 1b also shows the effects of parathyroid extract on constituents of the urine; notice the marked increase in phosphate concentration while urine calcium levels remain fairly constant. Notice also that this enhancement of phosphate excretion is associated with a fall in plasma phosphate levels.

QUESTION   If PTH acts solely to decrease phosphate levels in the plasma, what would be the effect on calcium plasma levels?

ANSWER   An increase, since the product of calcium and phosphate concentration is a constant.

---

* *The Open University (1971) S100* Science: A Foundation Course, *The Open University Press.*

Because of this response, for some years it was assumed that the primary action of parathyroid was to promote phosphate excretion by the kidney. (The details of this effect are not described here; you will learn more about the kidney in Unit 10.) The rise in serum calcium levels was assumed to be a secondary response resulting from lowered plasma phosphate levels. While it is now accepted that some of the observed changes in calcium levels *are* secondary, there is overwhelming evidence that parathyroid hormone has a direct effect on calcium: its release promotes the passage of calcium into the blood from bone.

A proportion of the calcium in bone, probably about 10 per cent, appears to be in equilibrium with the calcium in the blood. This proportion can be thought of as being freely available to maintain blood calcium levels; it is referred to as comprising the 'exchangeable bone', in distinction from the relatively inert 90 per cent.

exchangeable bone

Bone is composed of a tough organic matrix, strengthened by deposits of inorganic salts, principally calcium and phosphate. Despite its high inorganic content, bone is normally in a state of flux: cells called osteoblasts continually deposit it; other cells called osteoclasts continually absorb it. Normally, except in growing bones, the rates of deposition and absorption are equal, so the total mass of bone remains constant. When parathyroid tissue is transplanted in close proximity to bone, there is local absorption. Furthermore, following the removal of parathyroids in the rat (parathyroidectomy) the number of osteoclasts in bone diminishes, but increases when parathyroid extract is administered. Thus the changes in blood calcium may be a direct result of changes in the number of osteoclasts, induced by parathyroid hormone. An alternative theory suggests that parathyroid hormone promotes the metabolic activity of osteoclasts. An enhanced production of lactic and citric acids leads to small local changes in pH; this results in some of the previously insoluble calcium phosphate being brought into solution.

osteoblasts
osteoclasts

Thus the major effect of parathyroid hormone is to stimulate bone cells to free some of the calcium phosphate which was otherwise insoluble—it will not affect the 10 per cent or so that comprises the 'exchangeable bone'. The hormone does, however, act to a lesser extent to increase the rate of absorption of dietary calcium from the gut, and to promote the *retention* of calcium by the kidney.

QUESTION   The removal of the parathyroid glands results in a drop in plasma calcium levels. How would you account for this effect in terms of the mode of action of parathyroid hormone described above?

ANSWER   Parathyroidectomy results in reduced calcium absorption from bone, due to a reduction of parathyroid hormone levels.

If then, parathyroid hormone acts primarily to promote calcium resorption, what is the significance of its effect on phosphate excretion? Most probably the effect of the hormone on the kidney helps the disposal of phosphate liberated by increased resorption of bone. In addition, a drop in serum phosphate levels will reduce the rate of mineral deposition of bone; thus calcium levels will be maintained. In addition, the hormone has other effects mentioned above. It increases calcium retention in the kidney, so that *less* calcium is excreted (this effect is not always apparent, Fig. 1), and increases intestinal uptake. But what factors modify the release of parathyroid hormone?

PTH and bone

QUESTION   If parathyroid output were under feedback control, which chemical would modify its release?

ANSWER   Calcium, and possibly phosphate.

The intravenous injection of calcium causes a rapid fall in the concentration of parathyroid hormone in the blood; a reduction of blood calcium is followed by a sharp rise in parathyroid hormone content of the blood. In further experiments, low-calcium blood was perfused through an isolated thyroid/parathyroid preparation and the perfused fluid collected and injected into a parathyroid-ectomized animal.

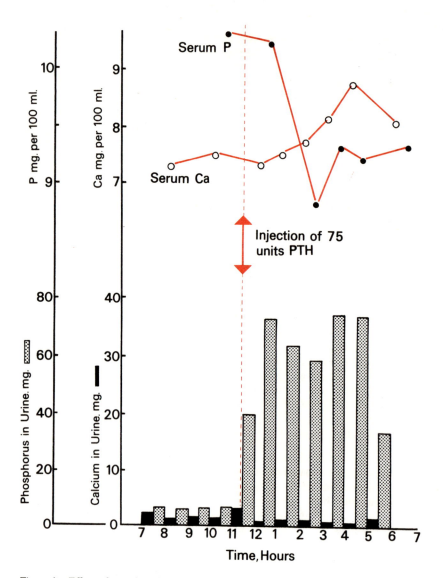

Figure 1 Effect of parathyroid extract on (a) serum levels of calcium and phosphorous and (b) urinary levels of calcium and phosphorus in a parathyroid deficient man.

QUESTION   What effect on serum calcium levels would you predict following the injection of the collected perfusion fluid?

ANSWER   An elevation of serum calcium levels, because lowered calcium levels appear to stimulate parathyroid hormone release.

This is, in fact, what happens. There is strong evidence that the level of calcium in the blood modifies parathyroid hormone release by a negative feedback. A fall in blood calcium results in parathyroid hormone release; an elevation of serum calcium produces an inhibition of parathyroid hormone release.

9.1.4   Vitamin D

PTH is not the only substance involved in the process of maintaining an adequate level of blood calcium. A disease called rickets has been recognised for many years, in which the bones of growing children fail to calcify. It is caused by a combination of poor diet and lack of sunlight; thus it is typically a disease of urban children in temperate climates.

rickets

The effect of the poor diet is, of course, that it provides too little calcium. For various reasons, calcium ions (Ca‡) are not easily absorbed by the gut even if plentifully available, and in addition other factors in the diet (for example phytic acid, present in wheat germ) may make some of the calcium completely insoluble. The absence of sunlight is relevant because ultra-violet light acts on

Ca absorption

6

steroids (e.g. 7-dihydrocholesterol) in the upper layers of the skin, and causes their breakdown into a physiologically active molecule called *calciferol*, or *vitamin D* (there are in fact a number of D vitamins now known). In furry animals the steroid is secreted on the hair, which is licked from time to time.

It appears that vitamin D acts in a way very similar to PTH, in that it promotes Ca absorption from the gut, and also assists in the mobilization of 'non-exchangeable' bone. However, there is now evidence which indicates that, contrary to earlier belief, calciferol acts differently from PTH on the kidney. In cases of calcium deficiency it can be shown that vitamin D causes *retention* of PO_4 by the kidney.

What is the effect of keeping a high blood phosphate level?

Calcium will tend to be forced out of solution, into the bones.

This may be the reason for the importance of vitamin D to growing bones; in effect PTH maintains an adequate *blood* calcium at the expense of the bones, whereas vitamin D may be a factor which tends to preserve the *bones* during prolonged calcium deficiency. Further work could reveal a very interesting situation of mixed synergism and antagonism.

9.1.5 Calcitonin

Quite recently, the results of several experiments have indicated that an additional regulatory hormone is involved in the maintenance of mammalian plasma calcium levels. This hormone, called *calcitonin*, acts in the opposite way to parathyroid hormone—it lowers blood calcium levels, i.e. it is a *hypocalcaemic* agent. If, for example, high-calcium blood is perfused through a thyroid/parathyroid gland preparation, and the perfused blood subsequently injected into other animals, there is a prompt fall in plasma calcium levels. Thus a high calcium level seems to release a hypocalcaemic agent.

calcitonin

QUESTION   Approximately thirty minutes after injection of the extract, the calcium returns to normal. What factors might account for this rapid return to normal calcium levels?

ANSWER   A drop in calcium levels, induced by calcitonin injection, might evoke parathyroid hormone release, which tends to elevate blood calcium.

In normal conditions, the level of blood calcium is mainly determined by parathyroid and calcitonin hormones. What is the significance of this dual control (often called a 'push-pull' mechanism) where two hormones act antagonistically in maintaining a constant level of a single substance?

push-pull

One clue to the normal function of these two hormones comes from the observation that the time taken to exert their maximum effects on blood calcium levels are quite distinctive. Calcitonin acts rapidly, achieving its maximum effects after only one hour. Parathyroid hormone has a more prolonged action—its greatest effects are apparent some three or four hours following its administration. It is likely that if calcium levels were maintained solely by parathyroid hormone, its prolonged action would result in marked oscillations of blood calcium concentration with occasional excessive (or 'overshoot') levels. In these conditions, calcitonin could play a useful role since its rapid hypocalcaemic action would tend rapidly to restore normal calcium levels.

What is known of the evolution of this hormone is also interesting. It has been known for many years that a small gland in the pharynx of fish, formed from epithelial tissue at the base of the last gill pouch, exerted some influence on calcium metabolism. This gland was called the *ultimobranchial gland*; you may note an analagous situation to the one described by Professor Barrington in the TV programme of Unit 8, the evolution of the thyroid. In adult mammals, the ultimobranchial glands are no longer separate, but incorporated into the thyroid gland. In various teleost fish, chickens and turkeys, extracts of the ultimobranchial gland produce a polypeptide with an hypocalcaemic action; it

ultimobranchial gland

appears to be calcitonin. Thus the calcitonin orginating from the thyroid in mammals may be secreted from cells derived from the ultimobranchial gland.

9.2 Blood Sugar

The concentration of glucose in the circulating blood (blood sugar level) is a matter of great physiological importance. This is because glucose is the major source of energy in the body and its level in the blood is a measure of its availability to the tissues: in the blood it may be *en route* from the gut to the tissues burning it, or from tissues acting as food stores to other tissues burning or storing it.

In Man, the level of glucose in the blood normally varies between 70 and 110 mg per 100 cm³ of blood. If it falls as low as 50 mg (*hypoglycaemia*) various disturbances such as loss of the power of concentration, cold sweating, shaking and nausea are felt. Below about 40 mg/100 cm³, convulsions may start, followed by coma; if the level is not rapidly raised, the coma may be fatal. Under some circumstances the level may rise as high as 180 mg, but at this level most individuals will have passed what is called the *renal threshold*, that is to say glucose begins to appear in the urine. Much above this level, coma may result, this time from *hyperglycaemia*. In both cases the coma is a result of effects on the brain: in hypoglycaemia it is largely an insufficiency of glucose to keep up brain cell metabolism; in hyperglycaemia the blood becomes very acid, which rapidly affects the brain cells. In either case, the level is clearly a matter of importance, and its regulation within the normal narrow limits is a matter of great physiological interest.

You have already considered one homeostatic mechanism operating on a constituent of the blood, Ca, but what makes the regulation of glucose level of particular interest as an example of hormonal co-ordination is that so many different factors may affect it. Blood sugar may tend to rise or fall for a number of totally different and unrelated reasons; it could be argued that a really efficient systems engineer would design the process so that the final regulatory path was the same, whatever the source of the demand for, or surplus of, blood sugar. However, on this view, it has to be admitted that, at a physiological level of organization anyway, the Designer moved in a mysterious way!

9.2.1 Maintenance of a constant blood sugar level following a meal

Immediately following the digestion and absorption of a meal containing carbohydrate, there will be a tendency for the level of blood sugar to rise sharply. The carbohydrate will be digested to monosaccharides (or sometimes disaccharides), a large proportion of which will be glucose, though others such as fructose may also be present, depending on the carbohydrate. Fats and proteins, though they may ultimately end up as blood sugar, will of course initially enter the bloodstream as fat droplets, fatty acids or amino acids, and therefore do not enter our calculations at this point.

It is not difficult to eat 250–300 g of carbohydrate at one sitting; however, normal blood level is 100 mg of glucose per 100 cm³ of blood, which is 1 g per litre, and an average figure for the blood volume of a man is 5 l (a woman 3·5 l). Thus the amount of glucose circulating in the blood at the start of a meal will be likely to be less than 5 g in a man and 3·5 g in a woman; yet over a period of 2–3 hours the circulation may be presented with anything up to a hundred times this amount.

It is apparent that there must be a mechanism which is both fast-acting and sufficiently widely dispersed to result in the storage of the excess glucose in a large number of cells; without such a mechanism, eating even an ounce of sugar would result in rapid coma. Figure 2 shows the effect on the level of blood glucose of eating 50 g of glucose. Clearly some mechanism is coming into play in less than half an hour, to counteract the effect of absorbing glucose through the gut wall.

The absorbed glucose will enter the circulation via the hepatic portal vein, which drains the blood supply to the gut, and pass directly to the liver before

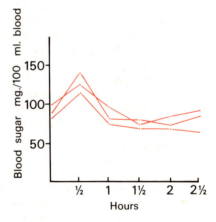

Figure 2 Effect on the level of blood glucose of three men of doses of 50 g of glucose taken by mouth.

being carried to the heart and round the rest of the circulation. The liver is a major store of carbohydrate, as the cells may hold large quantities of glycogen (see S100, Units 14, and 15–16), but its normal level of uptake of glucose (and other monosaccharides) from the portal blood does not approach the sort of increment we are discussing here.

If you give a glucose meal to an animal from which the pancreas has been removed, there is a catastrophic effect on the level of blood glucose—the renal threshold is rapidly passed and coma follows—unless the meal is small. The reason for this is known to be that the pancreas is the source of a hormone which depresses the level of blood sugar. The site of secretion is not the exocrine part of the gland (see Unit 4) responsible for the production of digestive enzymes, but separate groups of secretory cells occurring in little clumps in the pancreas. These are called 'the islets of Langerhans', and it is the cells within them that are responsible for the secretion of the hormone (Fig. 3). The hormone was first extracted in 1922 and called *insulin*; it is a protein, and when its detailed structure was finally completely deciphered by Sanger in the late 1950s, the work won him a Nobel prize. It was the first time the structure of a protein had been revealed in full.

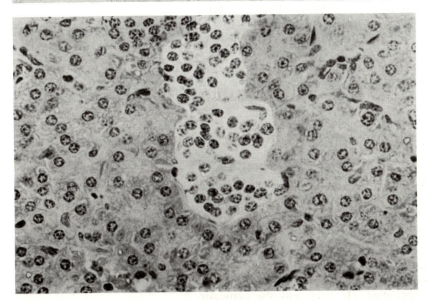

Figure 3a and b   Photomicrographs of islets of Langerhans within the pancreas.

In terms of the control system, there are strong similarities with what you know of parathyroid hormones. In the case of insulin, however, its release follows a *rise* in the glucose level of the blood supplying the cells (PTH is released following a fall in blood Ca). Insulin acts at a number of different points to reduce the level of the blood glucose; the result of insulin secretion is to accelerate the

depancreatized animal

islets of Langerhans

insulin

9

manufacture of glycogen from circulating glucose, particularly in muscle cells, but also to some extent in the liver.

Later in this Unit we discuss what little there is known of the details of how various hormones achieve their effects at the cellular level, but as this stage we will confine ourselves to mentioning the action in general terms.

Glucose from the blood must be transported across the muscle cell membrane and phosphorylated to form glucose-6-P before it can either be stored as glycogen or burnt by the cell. If you need to remind yourself of the glycolytic sequence, you should re-read the relevant part of S100, Unit 15.

muscle cells

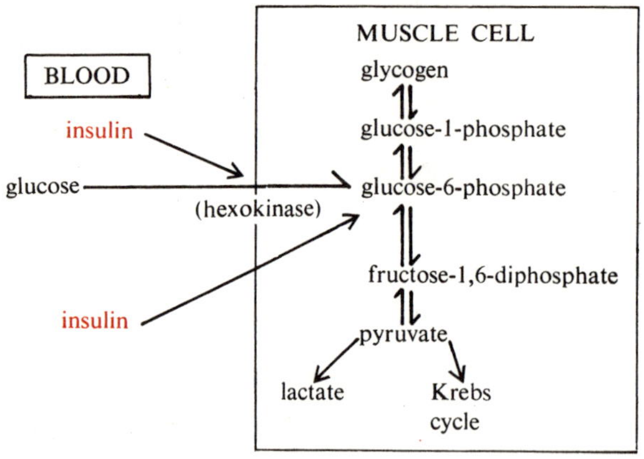

Figure 4 *Sites of action of insulin on glucose uptake by a muscle cell.*

It is possible that the processes of getting the glucose across the membrane and of phosphorylating it are actually linked, but nevertheless it is possible to demonstrate two separate sites of action of insulin near the point of entry of glucose to the muscle cells (Fig. 4). One is on the transport system across the cell membrane—insulin renders the membrane very much more permeable to glucose; and the other is on the enzymes of glucose-6-phosphate formation, including hexokinase.*

hexokinase

The first of these two effects does not apply to liver cells, gut cells, brain cells, blood cells or kidney cells; thus it seems rather specific for muscle tissue. Exactly what is happening at what we called the 'second site' is not entirely clear—though it is undoubtedly complicated. (Unfortunately, in this context, the study of insulin action is one of the most complex and confused areas of endocrinology.) First of all, the 'second site' is in fact many sites. Several enzymes that catalyse reactions in the glycolytic sequence are stimulated by insulin, with the result that glucose is phosphorylated faster and glycogen formation is increased.

Thus the overall picture suggests that insulin is having a two-step action on the uptake of glucose by the muscle cell (though this view is open to challenge), the first being to accelerate transport across the cell membrane, the second to increase the rate of phosphorylation and glycogen formation.

In liver cells, the situation is rather different. As we said above, insulin has no effect on the permeability of the cell to glucose (the cell membrane is in fact freely permeable to glucose), although again one of the rate-limiting steps here is the hexokinase–activated phosphorylation. (In liver cells the particular

liver cells

* *It is interesting to note that for many years most textbooks claimed that insulin acceler-ated the uptake of glucose by the liver—yet what evidence there was largely contradicted this. It is only the recent work on the second site of action of insulin, where it affects the rate of phosphorylation, that has provided evidence that insulin may indeed accelerate the uptake of glucose into the liver. Probably the liver of a mammal on a natural diet does not often take up glucose from the blood anyway; the high level of starch in the modern human diet accounts for the flood of glucose into the blood after a meal.*

hexokinase involved differs from the one in muscle cells, and is called *gluco-kinase*.) As we suggested in the case of muscle cells, it seems that insulin may accelerate this step; but the evidence is less clear for liver cells, and some workers still doubt if there is any *direct* effect by insulin on the uptake of glucose in this case.

glucokinase

Thus, in summary, following an inrush of glucose into the bloodstream and the beginning of a rise in blood sugar above about 100 mg per 100 cm³, the islets of Langerhans secrete (or increase their secretion of) insulin, which greatly accelerates the uptake of glucose by the muscles and liver, particularly the former. This results in the increased formation of glycogen, which is stored within the cells of these tissues. The release of insulin has been shown to correlate with variations in the blood sugar (of the dog) in the range of 40–600 mg/100cm³.*

A deficiency in the ability of the islet cells to secrete insulin results in the disease called *diabetes*, or more accurately *diabetes mellitus*, 'sugar diabetes'.

diabetes

QUESTION   If there is a partial insulin deficiency, what sort of symptoms would you expect to occur?

ANSWER   After a meal containing carbohydrate the blood sugar level will rise abnormally high and glucose will appear in the urine. Possibly also a hyperglycaemic coma will follow.

QUESTION   What might be the effect on the state of general vigour and muscle energy reserves?

ANSWER   Dietary carbohydrate will not enter the muscle cells at the proper rate, so their glycogen reserves will be low. (This may also apply to the liver.) In exercise, the muscle cells will not even be able to make use of the circulating glucose properly as its uptake will be slowed. Therefore, there will be muscular weakness and a good deal of muscular wasting. Valuable energy will be being excreted as urinary glucose.

QUESTION   What sort of treatment would seem reasonable?

ANSWER   1   Assessment of the degree of the deficiency in order to prescribe an *accurate* dosage of insulin (too much would cause a dangerous hypoglycaemia);
2   injection of an insulin supplement;
3   regulation of the dietary intake of carbohydrate.

Until now, insulin has had to be introduced into the body by injection; taking it by mouth has been ineffective.

Can you think why?

Insulin is a protein, and will not be absorbed whole; the molecule will be digested.

It is interesting to note that insulin secretion is triggered not only by a rise in blood glucose, but also by the secretion of the gastro-intestinal hormones such as secretin and pancreozymin (Unit 4). Thus insulin secretion may begin, at least to a small extent, as soon as a meal is taken, even before the blood sugar rises significantly.

* At this juncture we should emphasize one very important point about the action of insulin. In this Unit we are concerned mainly with the regulation of blood sugar, as an example of homeostasis; for this reason we have been considering only the homeostatic effects of insulin on glucose. However, insulin has many other important metabolic effects, some of them resulting from the fact that it acts quite generally to clear the blood of potential 'fuels'—for it causes the removal from the blood of not only glucose, but also amino acids, and lipids in the form of fatty acids and triglycerides.
These latter effects are every bit as important in the regulation of the animal's metabolism as are the effects on glucose; not only do they affect the animal's energy usage but, just as removal of glucose from the blood is associated with the build up of glycogen, so the removal of amino acids and lipids is associated with protein synthesis and the build up of fat deposits. Indeed, the cells of the fat depots are the other main group of cells besides muscle which can be shown to be very sensitive to insulin.

You may notice (Fig. 5) that after glucose absorption has finished, the blood levels may be a little lower than at the start. This is doubtless due to the presence on the muscle cell membranes of some 'residual' insulin. However, insulin is a very powerful hormone and it becomes bound to the surface of muscle cells, where it remains for some time, so it is surprising that the 'overshoot' effect is not marked much more.

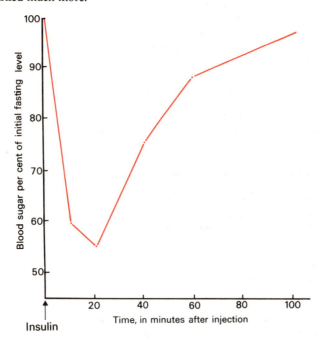

Figure 5 Effect on the level of blood glucose of a man of the injection of 0·1 unit of insulin per Kg of body weight.

QUESTION By analogy with the Ca and PTH situation, can you suggest any possible 'smoothing' mechanism?

ANSWER A quick-acting antagonistic hormone from a different source, released if the blood level begins to fall too low, analogous to calcitonin.

It has been known for forty years or more that the activity of insulin extracts could vary, and in particular that those prepared by the technique favoured in the United States were often less active than the European extracts.

It became apparent that some preparations contained traces of an insulin antagonist. This was isolated in 1952, and the structure of the molecule determined in 1956. It was called *glucagon* in 1924, when it was an unknown contaminant, and the name has remained. It is a polypeptide, a much smaller molecule than insulin, and very active.

glucagon

A detailed study of the islets (Fig. 3, p. 9) reveals that there are in fact three distinct types of secretory cell, which have been called the *α*, *β* and (by an unhappy mixing of alphabets) C cells. The origin of insulin is in the *β* cells. The *α* cells have been shown to be the source of glucagon; the function of the C cells is as yet unkown.

α and β cells

Once again, stimulation appears to be direct, in that a lowering of the sugar level of the blood supplying the islets results in the secretion of glucagon.*

---

* *This was not easy to demonstrate by direct methods twenty years ago—indeed, even using modern techniques, it is difficult to assay the amount of glucagon in circulating blood, as the amounts are small and it is rapidly destroyed by the liver. The technique used was a 'crossed circulation': the blood of a dog with hypoglycaemia (dog A) was circulated through the pancreas of a test dog (B) whose own pancreatic artery was clamped off; the pancreatic vein was left intact so that the blood of dog A went through the pancreas of B and into its general circulation. Although dog B had previously had normal blood sugar, a substance appeared in its blood which resulted in hyperglycaemia.*

The glucagon acts to increase blood sugar by accelerating the breakdown of liver glycogen to glucose-6-P, which is followed by dephosphorylation and release into the blood as glucose (Fig. 6).

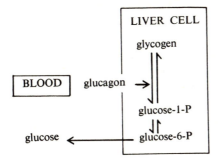

Figure 6   Site of action of glucagon on liver glycogen.

It does this by increasing the proportion of the enzyme *phosphorylase*, which catalyses the initial breakdown of glycogen to glucose-1-P. (Glucose-1-P and glucose-6-P will be in equilibrium, so that an increase in G-1-P will result in the production of more G-6-P.)

It appears that the phosphorylase which catalyses this reaction exists in two states: phosphorylase 'a' (active) and phosphorylase 'b' (inactive). These are in equilibrium, and glucagon acts to shift this equilibrium in favour of phosphorylase 'a' (Fig. 7).

action of glucagon

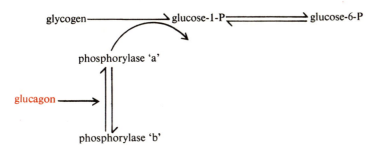

Figure 7   Apparent mode of action of glucagon on liver glycogen.

We shall return to this point with more of an explanation in Section 9.3 of this Unit. However, to summarize: glucagon acts to increase the phosphorylase-catalysed breakdown of liver glycogen into glucose-1-P, which results in the appearance of glucose in the blood.

The effect is rapid, 1 μg of glucagon injected into a man produces a rise in the blood sugar of 50 mg/100cm^3 within six minutes; the rise would probably be greater in a depancreatized man. (The rise produces a prompt compensatory secretion of insulin, also within six minutes, in an intact man.)

We said above that glucagon acted on liver glycogen reserves; it does not act on muscle glycogen, however. This is both an interesting and a physiologically important point. First, it demonstrates the remarkable specificity of some enzymes, because there must be some difference between the phosphorylase system which catalyses glycogen → glucose-1-P in muscle and that which catalyses it in liver cells *in the same animal*—otherwise the same glucagon would be bound to affect both systems. (It is, of course, possible that this difference is due to the location of the enzymes rather than to chemical differences —for example, the glucagon may be membrane-bound and the muscle phosphory-lase may be farther away from the membrane than is the liver phosphorylase system.) This enzyme specificity has the effect of making the action of the hormone at the cellular level highly specific, which leads us to the second point of interest.

The system of maintaining homeostasis of the blood sugar—by balancing the effects of a hormone that tends to push glucose into the muscle (insulin) with the effects of one that pulls glucose out of the liver (glucagon)—acts to promote the build up of muscle glycogen. Once the muscle glycogen is there, it will stay in the muscles, where it is needed to provide energy for physical work, rather than have increments removed again to maintain the blood sugar level. Thus the insulin/glucagon system acts rather like a hand-pump with valves: on the 'push' carbohydrate goes into the muscle, but on the 'pull' it comes out of the liver.

pump analogy

Thus we have in this sytem a homeostatic mechanism which will accommodate the influx of large amounts of sugar into the blood without correspondingly large changes in the level of circulating blood sugar; but it is also one which will effectively smooth out small changes in sugar levels, up or down, due to normal metabolic demand or other causes.

There are, however, other situations that also call for the regulation of the amount of circulating blood sugar.

9.2.2 Regulation of the blood sugar in exercise

There are times when the homeostatic problem will not be how to cope with a large and sudden inrush of blood sugar, but rather how to contain a large and sudden drain on it.

What common circumstances might lead to this heavy demand?

Exercise, particularly violent exercise.

Not only will there need to be a fast-acting, widespread mechanism to adjust to this demand, but there are circumstances when it may be very advantageous to the animal if it actually anticipates the demand. If the violent exercise is fighting, or fleeing from a hostile situation, there may well be an advantage in starting to mobilize the glycogen reserves before the blood sugar level has in fact fallen—a sort of pre-emptive homeostasis.

The scale on which demands may be made on the blood sugar can be judged when it is realized that in very vigorous exercise a man may burn the equivalent of 5 g of glucose in one minute.

Try to recall the average figure for the total amount of blood sugar in circulation at any one time.

About 5 g, or rather less.

Now, the muscles themselves will normally contain substantial reserves of glycogen, perhaps 300 g in all, so the load will not immediately and completely fall on the blood sugar. However, the muscles make very rapid use of the glucose in the capillaries as well as breaking down their intra-cellular glycogen (a process which may take a little time) and using other immediate energy stores within the cell. Furthermore, the process of withdrawing glucose to replace the lost reserves will begin immediately. Thus, clearly, drastic measures are called for to mobilize glycogen reserves as blood sugar if a disastrous hypoglycaemia is to be avoided.

Logically, which glycogen reserves would be best placed for this purpose?

Those in the liver cells. The muscle glycogen is already 'in the front line', and as you will see later, there are biochemical difficulties in using this as a source of blood sugar.

From what we have said earlier, this effect could be achieved by the rapid and large-scale release of glucagon, but it is not. We will consider the possible reasons for this a little farther on (p. 15).

Can you recall a hormone which is rapidly released in response to sudden environmental stress—in 'fight, flight or fright'?

Adrenalin (S100, Unit 18, and Unit 5 of this Course).

As you know, adrenalin causes a number of changes in the circulation which are important in vigorous activity. It also is very potent in accelerating the breakdown

adrenalin

of liver glycogen, which is then converted to blood glucose in the usual manner.*

adrenal medulla

The adrenalin released in quantity into the bloodstream comes from the medulla of the adrenal glands. Sympathetic nerve fibres run from the spinal cord to the adrenal medulla, where they make synaptic contact with cells which are derived from embryonic sympathetic nerve cells. The medulla cells are specialized for the secretion of massive amounts of adrenalin, rather than for the functional conduction of nerve impulses with the release of small amounts of adrenalin at their terminations, as would be normal for post-synaptic sympathetic nerve cells.

When adrenalin reaches the liver, it acts to mobilize glycogen by accelerating the phosphorylase-catalysed breakdown of glycogen to glucose-1-P. Thus it acts at precisely the same point as does glucagon, although it is an entirely different molecule.

QUESTION Can you think of any advantage accruing to an animal which can mobilize liver glycogen by means of adrenalin as compared to one which depends on glucagon release alone?

ANSWER Use of adrenalin means that the animal has linked the ability to increase its blood sugar to the nervous system, rather than having only a homeostatic device monitoring the existing blood levels. Thus it can 'anticipate' the demand for blood sugar or increase it for other reasons, if this is advantageous (see p. 14).

---

site of action of adrenalin

There is at least one important difference between the actions of adrenalin and glucagon. Whereas glucagon acts predominantly on liver glycogen, adrenalin acts equally on the phosphorylases of muscle and liver cells, so that glycogen is rapidly broken down in muscle cells as well, leading to an increase in the intracellular pool of glucose-6-P.

However, at this point we encounter another very interesting difference between muscle and liver cells. Whereas in liver cells the glucose-6-P is dephosphorylated by the enzyme glucose-6-phosphatase and then released into the blood as glucose, no such reaction takes place in muscle cells. In fact, the enzyme glucose-6-phosphatase is lacking in the membranes of muscle cells.

So once again we have the 'pump' and 'valve' analogy operating. Insulin 'pushes' sugar into the muscle, but the adrenalin 'pull' withdraws it only from the liver. Clearly, there has been an advantage, throughout the evolution of these mechanisms, in *not* supporting the blood sugar level directly at the expense of the muscles (Fig. 8, p. 16).

(In the longer term, muscle glycogen may contribute indirectly to the blood sugar, because pyruvic acid which is not burnt in the Krebs cycle may be converted to lactic acid and then diffuse into the bloodstream to be resynthesized later by the liver into liver glycogen.)

QUESTION If an animal is in, or entering into, an 'emergency' situation, the release of sugar into the blood is produced by adrenalin rather than glucagon. Can you think of any advantage to an animal in this situation in secreting a hormone which affects *both* liver and muscle glycogen?

ANSWER The liver glycogen will of course give rise to increased blood sugar, but the early breakdown of muscle glycogen will be an important preparation for vigorous muscular work.

---

* *The importance of the release of adrenalin into the general circulation of a mammal may lie mainly in this effect. Its effect on the arterioles of the peripheral circulation may also be very important, though in many cases the muscles of these vessels have a direct sympathetic innervation which will produce faster and more controlled results. Certainly, its effect on the heart rate is slow and uncontrolled compared with the results achieved by the release of minute amounts of adrenalin by the sympathetic nerve terminations directly on the heart muscle and nodes. There would seem to be no obvious biological advantage in replacing the precise, controlled, nervous regulation of the heart by the much less controlled effects of circulating adrenalin, which will not in any case reach the heart until after the nervous effect has been felt. Thus this action of the circulating adrenalin is probably a secondary one.*

15

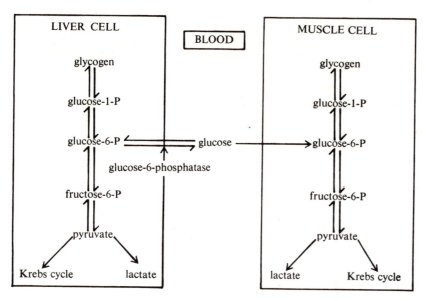

Figure 8   Relationship between blood glucose and the glucose-6-P in muscle cells and liver cells.

Thus, where the blood sugar is being raised in response to an insulin 'overshoot' and to 'resting' metabolic depletion, the hormone involved will usually be glucagon and the muscle glycogen will be untouched. Where the demand is drastic—and this is often associated with actual or anticipated vigorous muscular work— adrenalin will be involved, and both liver and muscle glycogen breakdown will occur, though the latter will not contribute directly to the blood sugar.

Finally, there is yet another interesting point of comparison between the actions of adrenalin and glucagon. Whilst glucagon antagonizes the action of insulin in its effect on the blood sugar level, it does not seem to have a direct effect upon insulin secretion itself. Adrenalin, on the other hand, has the additional effect of inhibiting insulin secretion by the β cells, thus enhancing its effect of raising the sugar level.

As you know, adrenalin release is brought about by the stimulation of the appropriate nerve fibres of the sympathetic nervous system. The main 'centres' of the sympathetic system appear to be located in the hypothalamus, indeed the hypothalmus has been called the 'head ganglion' of the sympathetic system (though you may feel that this is a rather limited view of hypothalamic function). These hypothalamic sympathetic 'centres' may be stimulated by higher nervous areas, as when fight or flight is anticipated, leading to adrenalin release. However, they may also be stimulated by lowered levels of sugar in the hypothalamic blood supply, so a large hypoglycaemia will lead directly to adrenalin release.

9.2.3   The relationship between glucagon and adrenalin in blood sugar regulation

This 'dualism' of hyperglycaemic factors is just one aspect of an intriguing question—how and why have these and other parallel hormonal mechanisms arisen? There is an irresistible temptation to speculate on the evolution of such mechanisms; but research in this field has to date been so limited as to establish only a few small islands of knowledge which must be joined by bridges of guesswork—a feat of engineering you should regard with caution.

Insulin occurs throughout the vertebrates, and is secreted by the islet cells of the pancreas in all except in the lamprey and its relatives, which have no pancreas. In the lamprey, there are 'follicle cells' in the gut wall, made up of what appear to be β cells, which were shown by Barrington in 1942 to be comparable to the islets in function. (You will recall that Professor Barrington spoke about research on the evolution of the thyroid gland in the television programme of Unit 8.) Insulin appears to play an important part in carbohydrate metabolism, even in the most primitive vertebrates; whether it is important in any of the invertebrate groups is not known.

It seems highly probable that the antagonistic mechanism will have evolved side by side with the insulin one; so it is interesting to consider which antagonist is the original or 'primitive' one—glucagon or adrenalin.

Glucagon might seem the most likely candidate in that it is produced by cells (α cells) with the same embryological origin as the insulin-producing β cells; the α cells are located in the same place, and apparently their secretion is also governed 'directly' by the level of sugar in the blood supplying them. ('Directly' is perhaps a rather misleading adverb—in this context it merely means 'as opposed to a mechanism involving a nervous reflex or trophic hormones'.) Furthermore, glucagon is a much more active hyperglycaemic agent than adrenalin, the latter being required in ten times the quantity to produce the same release of glucose from the liver.

Adrenalin on the other hand, with its secretion dependent on a nervous pathway involving the brain, could well be a newcomer to the metabolic scene. This would fit in with its physiological role in mammals, where it has overriding effects on blood sugar, achieved partly by inhibiting insulin release, but seen mostly only in emergency situations or in the cold (see p. 18). In this action, it is assisted by its effect on muscle glycogen, an effect not shared with glucagon.

On this view, the 'primitive' function of adrenalin is probably its action on the circulatory system, particularly the peripheral system, and the basic homeostatic antagonist to insulin is glucagon. Adrenalin might have acquired its metabolic importance during vertebrate evolution, or even earlier in a pre-vertebrate ancestor.

Obviously, it is of great interest to see what the pattern of blood sugar regulation is among the lower vertebrates, but unfortunately, as we said above, very little work has been done on this, and most of it dates back to the nineteen-twenties and thirties. However, we do know something. You are aware of the effects of adrenalin on the circulatory system of some fish (Unit 5, TV programme of Unit 6), and that it has been shown to be released in exercise. It has not been possible, however, to demonstrate any effect of adrenalin on liver glycogen, though it elevates blood sugar and lowers muscle glycogen. Insulin depresses teleost blood sugar, and this is true also of the lamprey, where Barrington showed that the 'follicles' referred to above reacted histologically to perfusion with a 10 per cent glucose solution in the same way as did other vertebrate cells, which seemed to suggest that insulin secretion was occurring. On the other hand, α cells have been described in the lamprey (though this has been challenged), and they certainly occur in teleost fish. Glucagon has been extracted from the islet cells of the catfish, *Ameiurus*, and hyperglycaemia follows the injection of glucagon into this species.

This evidence, scanty though it is, gives general support to the view of the evolution of adrenalin and glucagon outlined above. However, the picture becomes more difficult to interpret in other vertebrate groups. α cells are present in the anuran amphibians (e.g. frogs and toads), and these animals, like the teleosts investigated, are sensitive to both glucagon and insulin. However, the tailed amphibians (urodeles), such as the salamander, do not seem to have any α cells, only β ones. They are sensitive to insulin, but injection of glucagon apparently does *not* produce a hyperglycaemia. There seems to be no evidence one way or the other as to whether insulin is antagonized by adrenalin in this group.

The reptiles and the birds present even more enigmatic responses. They possess large numbers of α cells, and respond sensitively to glucagon. Their responses to insulin, however, are unlike those of other vertebrates in that there is relatively little depression of the blood sugar following insulin injection. It has been suggested that this is due to the very large number of α cells present—which may 'resist' the insulin by an antagonistic release of large amounts of glucagon— but the evidence for this is not convincing. Little or no information appears to be available at the moment as to the effects of adrenalin on the blood sugar of either reptiles or birds. Thus it is quite possible that reptiles and birds show the evolution of a blood-sugar regulating mechanism different from that of the surviving fishes, amphibia (except urodeles) and mammals.

Whilst it is most frustrating to lack the necessary information to be able to judge what the evolution of the mechanism really has been, the information we *do* have agrees quite well with the idea that the basic homeostatic mechanism has evolved as an insulin/glucagon balance. This does not, of course, preclude adrenalin from playing a part in normal homeostasis in the mammal—there may well be a low-level secretion of adrenalin tending to balance insulin secretion in addition to the emergency function; time will tell.

9.2.4   Effects of cold stress on blood sugar level

From various references in this Course (and in *S100*, Unit 18), you will be aware that hormones produced by the thyroid gland, thyroxin and tri-iodothyronine, are of the greatest importance in regulating the overall rate of metabolism, the 'basal metabolic rate'. In homoiotherms, the 'setting' of this basal rate determines the amount of heat made available to the body, and the activity of the thyroid gland is determined in part by climatic changes of the environment, acting via the hypothalamus (varying the release of thyroid stimulating hormone-releasing factor), which in turn effects the secretion by the pituitary of thyroid stimulating hormone.

thyroxin

The rate of secretion of thyroxin can be shown to be inversely related to the temperature; the effect of temperature change is not seen for some days, however, and the effect of circulating thyroxin on body temperature is also not immediate. Thus, varying the levels of thyroxin (and trio-iodothyronine) is a long-term adjustment—i.e. a method by which the homoiothermic animal adapts to seasonal variations in temperature. You can feel this adjustment subjectively; you may get out of bed on a March morning and think what a mild spring day it is, but if you get up to encounter precisely the same temperature in August you may be shocked by the cold, and feel extremely chilled.

The effect of increasing the thyroxin level in the blood appears to be to increase the rate at which blood sugar is taken up by the tissues, particularly the heart, skeletal muscles and liver, and the rate at which glucose enters the mitochondria of these tissues. With small doses, there is an increase in O_2 consumption, oxidative phosphorylation and heat production. Where rather large doses are given ($> 50\mu$ g/100 g per day), the process of phosphorylation becomes to some extent uncoupled from that of oxidation, so that when the glucose is 'burnt' in the mitochondria, a much higher proportion of the energy is dissipated as heat, rather than forming ATP for example. (These effects are possibly secondary in the sense that the primary action of the thyroid hormones is probably to influence the production of the enzymes involved.) Increased thyroid activity therefore tends to lower the blood sugar level, which will have to be maintained by increases in the diet or by the consumption of internal food stores such as the fat depots. The sugar level is kept up by the mechanisms we have already discussed, rather than by a specific thyroxin antagonist.

There are, of course, many situations where an immediate metabolic response to cold is necessary; clearly a homoiothermic animal cannot afford to cool down for several days after encountering a sudden drop in temperature. There are behavioural responses to cold, including shivering for example, but such responses have a number of disadvantages and are not always adequate. A rapid and effective metabolic response to a fall in blood temperature is produced by the secretion of adrenalin. This appears to follow quite a small drop in blood temperature, monitored in the hypothalamus, but is not accompanied by all the other 'emergency' responses of generalized sympathetic stimulation, such as sweating or dilation of the pupils of the eyes, though peripheral vasoconstriction and cardio-acceleration may follow the adrenalin release. There is also evidence that adrenalin release may begin before a fall in blood temperature occurs, as a result of nervous inputs to the hypothalamus from cold-receptors in the skin.

The effect of this adrenalin release is, of course, to raise the blood sugar above the normal level, at the expense of liver glycogen, and to increase the breakdown of glycogen to glucose-6-phosphate within the muscle cells. This increase in the 'pool' of available glucose has the effect of increasing the rate of carbohydrate metabolism and thus heat production; there does not appear to be any 'uncoupling' of oxidative phosphorylation. The process appears to be a very wasteful way of using food to keep warm, and seems only to be a short term expedient; if the cold situation persists, the process is supplanted by increased thyroxin production.

9.2.5 Production of blood sugar to meet the needs of the lactating mammary gland

One very large drain on the circulating blood sugar can be the production of milk by the mammary glands of female mammals. Milk contains sugar, in the form of *lactose*, a disaccharide composed of a glucose molecule joined to a galactose molecule; the galactose itself being formed from glucose (Fig. 9).

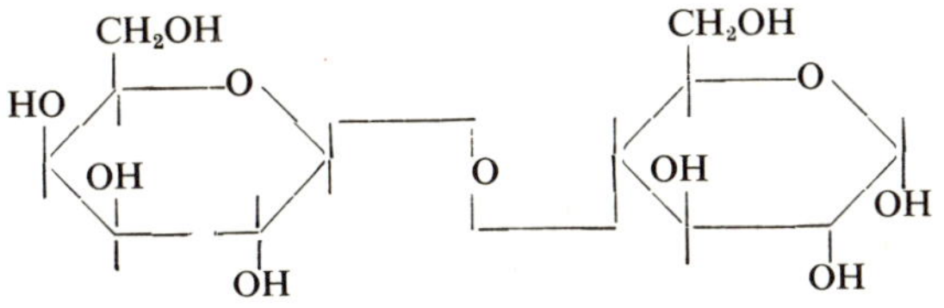

Figure 9   Structure of lactose molecule.

Depending on the mammal concerned, there may be 50–80 g l^{-1} of lactose in milk; in addition large amounts of energy are required for the production of the milk, so that in all something like 120 g of glucose are required for the production of 1 l of milk in cattle, and rather more in women, whose milk has a much higher lactose content.

(The hormonal control of the development of the mammary gland was mentioned in passing in Unit 8. The part played by hormones in glandular development and in the production of milk is both interesting and important; but as it is of only indirect relevance to this discussion we have included a brief note on the subject as Appendix 1.).

It is clear that the demands on the blood sugar will be very high; a dairy cow in milk may produce 23 l a day and even the production of 1 l by a woman will require some 130 g of glucose. (Recall how much glucose might be circulating in the blood of an average woman at any one time.) In the case of the dairy cow, this represents a major part of the energy available to it in its normal diet. In the face of a demand of this size from the mammary gland, it is obvious that much of the process of blood sugar regulation will in reality be simply blood sugar production and its subsequent transfer into the mammary gland cells.

milk secretion

QUESTION   Which, if any, of the hormones that we have described as involved in blood sugar regulation would you consider is likely to play a major part in maintaining the blood glucose during lactation?

ANSWER   None would seem ideal. *Glucagon* would tend to maintain the level if it were lowered below normal by the mammary gland, but only at the expense of liver glycogen. There are doubts as to the scale on which glucagon can normally be released to accelerate blood sugar production during exercise, and these doubts would be relevant here. Glucagon is almost certainly a component of a fine adjustment mechanism, at least in mammals.

Insulin would be inappropriate as it 'pushes' sugar into the muscles, whereas clearly the gland will need to have preference.
Adrenalin would have the desired effect on the blood sugar, but there would be severe drawbacks to the high adrenalin levels which would be needed. First, it causes peripheral vasoconstriction, and the gland is particularly sensitive to this—if you frighten a lactating cow, the blood flow through the udder may be reduced by 75 per cent, severely reducing milk secretion. Secondly, as we have seen above, a large amount of the blood sugar would go towards unnecessary heat production, which would be quite the wrong effect. The process of preparing animals for lactation is sometimes called 'steaming-up', but this is not meant literally!
Thyroxin, though important in lactation (see Appendix 1) will not elevate the blood sugar.
Thus it appears that some other hormonal mechanism would be more appropriate; the nature and source of this first became apparent following study of the effects on milk production of disease of the adrenal cortex.*

adrenal cortex

---

* The adrenal cortex is the outer or cortical layers of the adrenal gland. The inner or medullary region secretes adrenalin.

If the adrenal cortex is destroyed by disease or experimental procedures, milk secretion continues, but at only a few per cent of the normal rate. The adrenal cortex is known to be the source of a number of active steroid hormones, including small amounts of progesterone, androgens and oestrogens. In addition there are two major groups of steroids which are often called the *glucocorticoids* and the *mineralocorticoids*.

Examples of a glucocorticoid (*hydrocortisone*) and a mineralocorticoid (*aldosterone*) are given in Figures 10 and 11.

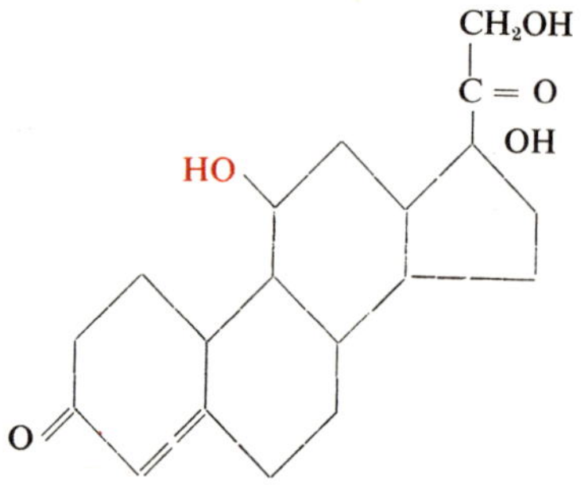

Hydrocortisone

Aldosterone

Figure 10   Structure of hydrocortisone.   Figure 11   Structure of aldosterone

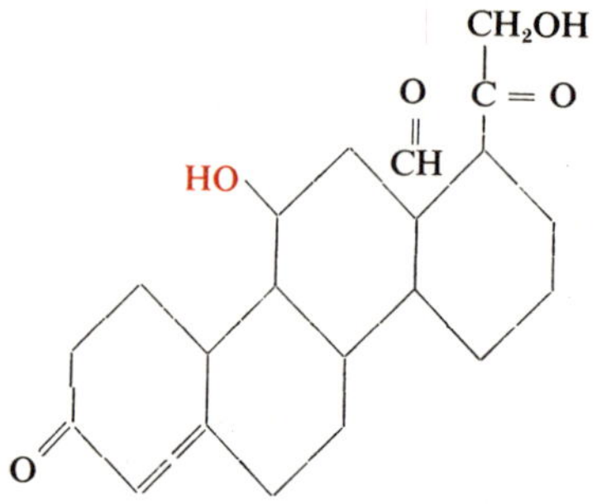

These names were given to the groups when it was believed that the former exerted their effects mainly on carbohydrate metabolism, and the latter on electrolyte balance. Those molecules with an oxygen of hydroxyl group on the C_{11} position were thought to be important in carbohydrate metabolism, but not in electrolyte balance. As you can see in Figure 11, aldosterone, one of the most important hormones in the control of electrolyte excretion, is an exception to that rule. It is now also known that almost all of the hormones in either group are active both in carbohydrate and in electrolyte metabolism; the distinction is a question of degree: for example, aldosterone is far more active in the latter field, and hydrocortisone in the former.

The adrenal corticoids are probably important in lactation for three different reasons. First, the mineralocorticoids may be essential for the large fluid and ionic movements involved (see Unit 10); secondly, there may be a direct effect by the glucocorticoids on the metabolism of the mammary gland cells and; thirdly, the glucocorticoids play a crucial role in the supply of blood sugar to the gland.

The glucocorticoids act in a number of ways which affect the blood sugar level.

1   They act antagonistically to insulin in that they *reduce* the uptake of glucose by the muscles, possibly by reducing the activity of the hexokinase reaction at the muscle cell membrane.

2   They act vigorously to increase protein breakdown in the muscle and connective tissue. The amino acids thus released are deaminated in the liver, and the carbon skeletons built up into liver glycogen, several of the enzymes involved in the latter process being activated by glucocorticoids.

3   They act to accelerate the breakdown of fatty tissue to glycerol and fatty acids, which also end up as liver glycogen.

Thus the general effects of the glucocorticoids are that they raise blood sugar by reducing glucose-consumption of the muscles, and produce a very large increase in liver glycogen at the expense of body protein and fat reserves. This situation is then coupled with the very high consumption of blood sugar by the mammary glands which will result in the circulatory sugar being replaced both from the diet and the liver glycogen. In effect, therefore, a cow lactating at a really high rate will be turning its dietary foodstuffs, fat reserves and some of its muscles (via liver glycogen) into milk.*

It is not altogether surprising that sometimes dairy cows give the impression of being composed of nothing but udder, bone and sorrow.

The control of glucocorticoid secretion is maintained by a trophic hormone from the anterior pituitary, a pattern with which you should now be thoroughly familiar! This hormone, a polypeptide, is called adrenocorticotrophic hormone (ACTH), and its release is in turn dependent on the descent of a releasing factor (corticotrophin releasing hormone, CRH) from the hypothalamus. There is a fast-acting negative feedback relationship between CRH and the circulating glucocorticoids; but sundry nervous stimuli, including stress of various kinds, may override this and increase CRH release, thus increasing the level of glucocorticoids in the blood.

ACTH

CRH

The factor that causes the increased release of CRH in lactation is not yet known, but it may well be linked to the suckling reflexes mentioned in Appendix 1.

Finally, a note of caution. Glucocorticoids play a part of the greatest importance in the metabolism of the animal, quite unconnected with their role in lactation. We have chosen to look at this one narrow aspect of glucocorticoid function for the same reasons as we confined our interest in the action of insulin to its effect on glucose in the blood—we are working to a very limited brief. Indeed, we are adopting a similarly limited view of the action of hormones in lactation; for example, although it is not clear what part insulin may play (if any) in the entry of glucose to the lactating gland, it is known that insulin *does* play a part in the transport of lipids from the blood into the gland and ultimately into the milk.

9.2.6 Summary of Section 9.2

In this Section we have seen a number of the hormonal mechanisms involved in maintaining the level of circulating blood sugar within the narrow limits (say 70–110 mg/100cm^3) necessary for the proper functioning of the body.

This level is maintained despite factors which vigorously oppose homeostasis; the ways in which homeostasis is, nevertheless, maintained are particularly interesting from an evolutionary as well as a physiological viewpoint. There is a 'push–pull' mechanism in the insulin/glucagon relationship which might seem logically to be sufficient to keep the blood level constant. In the event, however, the movements of sugar in and out of the blood may be determined by different hormones, depending on the nature of the 'threat' to the homeostasis. Whereas the sudden influx of sugar from the gut into the blood is 'damped down' by the insulin/glucagon mechanism, the sudden large demand presented by exercise involves a different antagonist to insulin—namely adrenalin. Where it is advantageous to generate increased heat, this can be done by increasing sugar consumption in the tissues (and thus its withdrawal from the blood) following increased thyroxin release; there is also an effective device for the short-term or 'emergency' production of heat, which involves speeding carbohydrate metabolism by elevating the blood sugar by adrenalin release. On the other hand, the large demands on the blood sugar made by the lactating mammary gland are met, in part at least, by the increased secretion of glucocorticoids such as hydrocortisone from the adrenal cortex.

The control mechanisms for integration of these responses vary considerably. Some general schemes are offered in diagrammatic form in Figure 12 (p. 22). Do you consider that these form a valid analysis of the systems involved?

* In the longer term, the effect of glucorticoids on the breakdown of body protein into free amino acids accelerates the manufacture of new protein. In the lactating animal, much of this new protein will be milk proteins, e.g. casein.

21

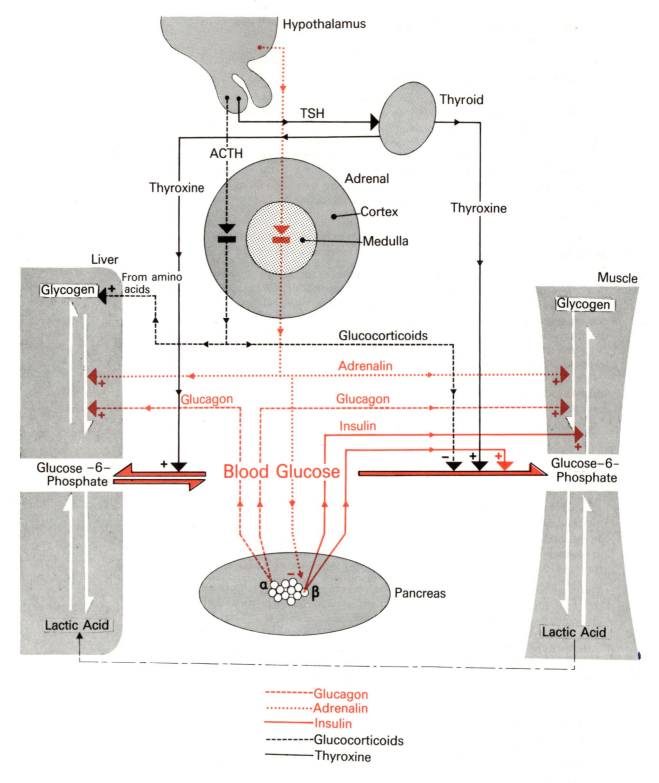

Figure 12 *Summary diagram of hormonal control of the blood sugar.*

9.3 The Actions of Hormones within the Cell

So far in this Unit we have concentrated on the effects of hormone systems on the organism as a whole, or on major tissues; we have identified the site of action mostly only as far as mentioning which tissues are involved, or occasionally which enzyme.

However, this stops far short of telling us *how* they produce their effects within the cell, or why a particular hormone will affect one cell but not another similar one—for example, the way in which testosterone stimulates some hair follicles but not others. The resolution of how hormones elicit responses from such specific targets is an exciting area of modern cell physiology.

In general terms, it is a problem of communication at the cellular level; communication requires that there be recognition and specificity. How is the hormone recognized by the appropriate target cells and how does it modify the activity of these cells? First consider the cell itself. You will remember from *S100* that a living cell establishes a dynamic relationship with its environment, and nutrients are exchanged across the cell membrane. The cell surface is in fact an extremely important control site for many cellular processes, and it is here that an examination of such a cellular communication system should begin.

Most hormones act on specific target cells; within these cells there are specific receptor sites, often on the cell membrane. The binding of a hormone molecule to such a site is held to be the first step in the body's response to that hormone and is the basis for recognition and specificity at the cellular level. But not all hormones bind to the cell surface; the steroids, for example, pass through the cell membrane and bind to receptor sites in the cytoplasm. However, such receptor sites, whether on the cell membrane or not, are thought to be proteins and the specificity of binding is thought to be analogous to the binding of a substrate to the active centre of an enzyme (refer to *S100* and the Biochemistry Course, S2–1, Unit 2).

Consider those hormones which initiate their effects at the cell membrane— what is the next step in the sequence of events? One of the earliest detectable biochemical events is an increased production inside the cell of a small nucleotide, *adenosine 3′ 5′ cyclic-AMP* (cyclic-AMP). Recognition of the physiological importance of this small molecule, and of its wide distribution and catholic functions, dates from work showing that cyclic-AMP mediates the hyperglycaemic effects of both glucagon and adrenalin.

cyclic—AMP

This finding has been extended to a wide variety of hormones and other biologically active agents, primarily on the basis of positive qualitative, quantitative and temporal correlations between the effects of hormones, cyclic-AMP levels and physiological response of the whole organism.

Following administration of these hormones, there is an increase in the activity of an enzyme of the plasma membrane, *adenyl cyclase*, which catalyses the conversion of ATP to cyclic-AMP. Moreover, there is a very complex relationship between the hormone-receptor protein and the adenyl cyclase, such that when the hormone binds to the receptor on the outside of the membrane this results in a conversion of the adenyl cyclase on the inside of the membrane from an 'inactive' to an 'active' form. The exact physico-chemical mechanism involved is not well understood and anyway need not concern us here. The beauty of the concept is that it provides us with an insight into how an extra-cellular signal can initiate important events inside a cell and thereby alter the direction of cell activity. Another important aspect of this kind of biological communication is taken account of by this model: given that hormones are effective at very low physiological concentrations there is a need for some means of amplification. A limited event on the outside of a cell puts in train processes which produce large amounts of cyclic-AMP, which can then affect a number of cellular activities over a prolonged period of time.

adenyl cyclase

Sutherland, an American physiologist who was awarded the Nobel Prize in 1971, has crystallized this into what has come to be called the *second messenger hypothesis*. The extra-cellular 'first messenger' (such as a hormone) promotes the amplified production of cyclic-AMP; the 'second messenger' and subsequent events are responses to this raised intra-cellular level of cyclic-AMP.

second messenger

Let us consider further how cyclic-AMP modulates cellular activity. You should recall that breakdown of glycogen is an important element in the control of blood sugar level. The action of cyclic-AMP was first unravelled in the phosphorylase enzyme system that breaks down glycogen in the liver. Cyclic-AMP activates a *kinase* (a type of enzyme that transfers a phosphate group), which converts an inactive *phosphorylase kinase* to an active phosphorylase kinase, which in turn

* *The Open University* (1972) *S2–1*, Biochemistry: A Second Level Course, *The Open University Press.*

converts *glycogen phosphorylase* from an inactive to an active form. Moreover, it seems that the same protein kinase inactivates the enzyme system synthesizing glycogen. The actions of the polypeptide hormone glucagon and the amine adrenalin have been interpreted in these terms. The complex sequence of events is best seen in Figure 13.

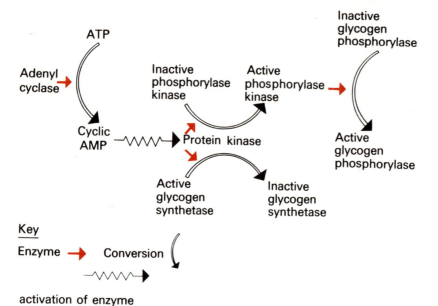

Figure 13   Action of cyclic-AMP on the breakdown of glycogen in the liver.

The diagram shows how cyclic-AMP, by activating one enzyme, can produce a series of reactions which act in an integrated fashion to promote glycogen breakdown and slow down its rate of synthesis. There is a good deal of evidence now to suggest that the first action of cyclic-AMP is generally to activate protein kinases. These kinases have been found in nearly all cells in a wide variety of groups from bacteria to mammals. Thus the general mechanism of action of these hormones acting on plasma membrane receptors might be represented as in Figure 14.

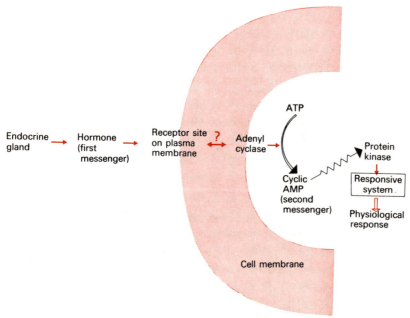

Figure 14   A generalized view of the action of some hormones on the cell.

In a general model such as this, the *specificity* of hormone action resides in the hormone/receptor interaction and any stereochemical constraints placed upon it. This is not always perfectly exclusive, indeed, some polypeptide hormones such as melanin-stimulating hormone (MSH) (a pituitary hormone which stimulates the dispersion of pigment granules in cells called melanocytes) and ACTH share

specificity

24

common sequences of amino acids; and ACTH also has some melanocyte-stimulating activity. This may indicate evolutionary duplication of the gene for MSH and subsequent divergence resulting in a new hormone with an adaptive relationship with a new target, the adrenal cortex. An important point that emerges from this is that no specificity resides in the cyclic-AMP system as such; the response of any given cell, such as a melanocyte, to ACTH will be appropriate merely as a function of the reaction of the unique set of enzymes of that cell to the altered intracellular cyclic-AMP levels.

Polypeptide hormones, such as vasopressin (see Unit 10), ACTH, glucagon, hypothalamic releasing factors and MSH, seem in general to fit this model, as do the hormones metabolically derived from amino acids, such as adrenalin and other amines, thyroxin and even some auxins (plant hormones).

One important polypeptide hormone which does not fit within the generalization is insulin, which, as you will remember, acts antagonistically to glucagon. According to the simple model, we would therefore expect it to *inhibit* adenyl cyclase. In fact this does not seem to be the case generally, although in a few situations insulin does result in a fall in the intra-cellular concentration of cyclic-AMP—this may be partly due to an increase in the activity of the enzyme which destroys cyclic–AMP, *phosphodiesterase*. But we have as yet no satisfactory explanation in biochemical terms of the mechanism of action of insulin. However, there are specific receptors for insulin on the plasma membrane of insulin-sensitive cells, and insulin can increase the permeability of muscle cell membranes to glucose. Further understanding of the events involved in its action must await more research.

phosphodiesterase

Unlike the polypeptide hormones and amines such as adrenalin, the steroid hormones do not seem to modulate the existing enzymes of the cell in this way, but are especially concerned with protein synthesis; they alter rates of protein synthesis and sometimes induce the synthesis of new proteins.

As mentioned before, the steroids pass through the cell membrane. When uterine cells are incubated with radioactively labelled oestradiol and then are disrupted and fractionated into subcellular components (a technique you may recall from *S100*), a highly specific protein-binding site can be demonstrated in the cell cytoplasm. After a short time the oestradiol–receptor complex is transferred from the cytoplasm and concentrated in the nucleus. Similar binding and transfer systems have been found for progesterone and testosterone, but the mechanisms underlying them are not well understood and it remains to be seen if, and then just how, cyclic-AMP is involved.

Specificity can be demonstrated in this system too. If an oestradiol–receptor complex and testosterone–receptor complex are incubated with nuclei from a variety of tissues, the former is bound preferentially by the nuclei of uterine cells and the latter by nuclei from cells of the testes and prostate gland. This is a promising area of research, as it allows investigators to 'map' target cells in different regions, e.g. oestradiol target cells are being found in various brain regions. These no doubt will ultimately be related to the role of oestrogens in modulating sexual behaviour.

But how can one hormone produce differeng responses in different cell types? This depends on the state of the cell itself; the nucleus seems to be the important site. After entering the nucleus, the hormones have been shown to bind to the chromosomes, or rather to certain acidic proteins associated with the DNA. Following this binding, there is an increase in RNA synthesis and, a little later, an increase of protein synthetic activity in the cytoplasm. The precise details of how protein synthesis is controlled are beyond our scope here, but there are several points at which control can occur: e.g. the rate of synthesis, by RNA polymers, of the various classes of RNA in the nucleus; or the translation process at the ribosomes in the cytoplasm. We can make no generalization at this stage as to how the steroids act. The intriguing thing is that cyclic-AMP-activated protein kinases have been shown to play a role in control at these various levels. But, at this time, understanding of the relationship of such processes to hormone action, the activation of genes and the control of protein synthesis is only indirect and tentative.

RNA synthesis

So far as the steroid hormones and their interaction with the cyclic-AMP system are concerned then, we are faced with many indirect and direct effects. For example, there is a growing body of evidence that oestrogen can raise cyclic-AMP levels in uterine cell cytoplasm indirectly, by promoting an amine stimulation of adenyl cyclase, but the precise molecular mechanism remains unclear. There are also several reports of activation of membrane-bound adenyl cyclases, e.g. by progesterone in chick oviduct, and the variation in female rat brain adenyl cyclase at different times in the oestrous cycle. But such data, derived from *in vivo* experiments, are extremely difficult to interpret.

There are also examples of polypeptide hormones which in certain cells have an effect on protein synthesis, as for example the induction of milk proteins by prolactin in differentiating mammary gland cells. Growth hormone also has an effect on protein synthesis amongst a number of other effects; for example, it results in an increase in cyclic-AMP content in certain cells and this may be mediated by an increased rate of synthesis of a protein component of the adenyl cyclase system itself. Such effects of growth hormone depend on the synergistic actions of a variety of other hormones, some of them steroids. Growth hormone also illustrates another dimension of the problem, for cyclic-AMP may be involved in a process that regulates the release of growth hormone from the pituitary.

We have uncovered here a range of problems pertaining to protein synthesis and the induction of enzymes, changes in cytoplasmic adenyl cyclase systems, interactions with other hormones and the role of cyclic-AMP and its related enzyme systems in the secretion of hormones. It is clear that the mechanism of action of some hormones is poorly understood and this is compounded when considering the co-ordinated response of whole populations of cells in a physiological context where hormones interact to produce their varied effects.

Nevertheless, there is some value in keeping in mind the broad distinctions between steroid hormones and those having plasma membrane receptors. It is also important to note that the cyclic-AMP/protein-kinase system crops up again and again: it is involved in nuclear metabolic events, where it may be important in influencing gene action; it modulates the activity of existing enzymes and mediates changes in membrane structure relevant to their physiological function. Given that such a small, ubiquitous, molecular modulator can be responsive to extra-cellular signals, such as hormones, and is found in all groups of organisms from bacteria to mammals, it probably has a very long evolutionary history as part of a cell-to-cell communication system. It is interesting that a similar adenyl-cyclase/protein-kinase system has now been implicated in the process of synaptic transmission.

This supports the suggestion that the hormonal and nervous co-ordinating mechanisms in higher animals, which traditionally are treated separately, represent an evolutionary divergence from a common cell-communication system which in its essence—if not in its ramifications—is subtle and elegantly simple.

Appendix I (White)   Hormones and Lactation

Clearly, a detailed account of lactation would be out of place in this Unit, but the process does provide an interesting illustration of the way in which very different types of hormonal mechanism may be employed in the different stages of a complex physiological event, and for this reason is worth a very brief note.

It is possible to consider the hormone patterns as falling into three main phases: those involved in the development of the gland in pregnancy, until it is in a state where it is ready to secrete; those involved in regulating the production and secretion of milk; and those involved in milk 'let-down' in response to suckling. There is, of course, a certain amount of overlap in these mechanisms.

You may recall from Unit 8 that the development of the gland in pregnancy provides an example of the synergistic action of oestrogen and progesterone. Oestrogen stimulates the rapid growth of blood vessels throughout the gland, increases the deposition of fat and causes the milk ducts to grow and branch inwards from the nipple. Normal, physiological doses of oestrogen, however, are not very effective in promoting the development of the secretory alveoli, the walls of which actually produce the milk. Alveolar development proceeds extensively when stimulated by rising levels of progesterone acting on the oestrogen-primed gland. Even when both duct and alveolar development have reached a high level, however, the ability to secrete milk may not be achieved. This depends on the action of the pituitary hormone, prolactin (once also known as luteotrophic hormone, LTH, from its action in causing progesterone secretion by the corpus luteum of the rat and mouse). By the end of pregnancy the developed gland is under the influence of prolactin, and might be expected to be able to secrete milk; however, it appears to be inhibited by the high levels of circulating oestrogen and progesterone (the former mainly from the placenta, the latter from both the placenta and the corpus luteum in those species which retain the corpus luteum until the end of pregnancy). Thus, although oestrogen + progesterone are essential for the development of the gland, if present in high levels they inhibit milk secretion.

After parturition, the progesterone level falls very low indeed, and the oestrogen falls to a modest 'base level'. This enables milk secretion to commence, though for the first few days a clear proteinous liquid called *colostrum* is produced instead. (Colostrum is important to species which have a placenta impermeable to antibodies, as it is the main route by which the young can acquire temporary immunity to disease. Instead of receiving the maternal antibodies through the placenta whilst still in the uterus—as is the case in man, for example—they absorb them through the gut after drinking colostrum. It is a remarkable process, as it involves a special adaptation of the gut, lasting only a few days, so that the maternal antibodies can be absorbed whole and undigested.) After a few hours or days, depending on the species, milk secretion gets underway. A moderate level of oestrogen stimulates milk secretion, but a high level inhibits it, as does the addition of progesterone to the system.

A great many hormones are necessary to maintain lactation, partly because of the enormous metabolic load it involves, and partly perhaps because of the high rate of renewal of the secretory epithelium of the alveoli. Thus a good level of thyroxin must be kept up (thyroidectomy results in a 90 per cent reduction in milk flow); PTH is necessary, probably because of the large amounts of calcium involved, and so are glucocorticoids (see Section 9.2.5), and a high level of prolactin. Prolactin may be crucial for the actual mechanism of secretion, though it also has important metabolic effects in the liver. We have already mentioned that a low level of oestrogen is desirable, and earlier in the Unit we said that insulin plays an important part in the uptake of lipids into the gland.

When the milk has been secreted, it lies in the alveoli; in the case of mammals with a large space (the 'cistern') just inside the nipple (e.g. cow and goat), about a third of the milk at any one time may be held there, but animals without a cistern hold very little in the ducts themselves. This means that when the young suckle, they can get very little milk by suction alone.

However, the process of suckling on the nipple (also the kneading or nuzzling of the gland which you may have seen the young of many mammals do) results

ducts

alveoli

prolactin

oestrogen and milk secretion

colostrum

27

in the initiation of a neurendocrine reflex. Sensory nerves from the gland, mostly in or around the nipple, carry impulses to the hypothalamus, which are relayed to the *posterior lobe* of the pituitary. Neurosecretory cells in the posterior lobe are then stimulated to release the hormone *oxytocin* (see ADH secretion in Unit 10), which travels around the circulation; when it reaches the aveoli of the mammary gland, it causes them to constrict (the epithelium itself is contractile and is called *myoepithelium* for this reason). This forces out the milk, a process which is called milk 'let-down'. Thus milk ejection is an entirely separate affair from milk production. Suckling does plays a part in the maintenance of lactation, however, as the regular sensory stimulation of suckling acts on the anterior pituitary on a long-term basis, to keep up the secretion of prolactin, and it also stimulates the thirst centres in the hypothalamus to increase the intake of water.

posterior lobe
oxytocin

myoepithelium

The process of milk let-down is easily interfered with. Anger or anxiety will block the secretion of oxytocin, and prevent an adequate let-down of milk for the child or animal. Nursing mothers and milking cows must be humoured. (It is not uncommon to find that the mothers of unwanted babies are physiologically unable to breast-feed them.) Any stimulus which is strong enough to cause sympathetic excitation will inhibit the blood flow to the gland (Section 9.2.5) by adrenalin release, and this may interfere with the manufacture of the milk, and also prevent the oxytocin reaching the gland.

This brief outline may enable you to pursue this aspect of reproductive physiology more easily on your own if you so wish; we hope it also gives you an idea of the sort of hormonal integration which may be involved in a major physiological event such as lactation.

Acknowledgements

Grateful acknowledgement is made to the following sources for material used in this unit:

Fig. 1 Williams and Wilkins Co. for F. Albright and E. C. Reifenstein, *Parathyroid glands and metabolic bone disease*, 1948; *Figs. 2 and 4* E. and S. Livingstone Ltd. for G. Bell, J. Davidson and H. Scarborough, *Textbook of Physiology and Biochemistry*, 1961.

Self-assessment Questions

Section 9.1

SAQ 1 (*Objective 10*) Sometimes a growth or tumour may develop on the parathyroid gland, with the result that large amounts of PTH are manufactured and released into the blood, giving a permanently elevated level of PTH. Where this situation lasts for many months, what effect do you think it is likely to have on:

(a) the level of Ca in the blood;

(b) the constitution of the bones;

(c) the levels of Ca and PO_4 excreted in the urine?

You can assume that the thyroid will not be capable of producing enough calcitonin to counteract the abnormal amount of PTH produced by a substantial growth of this kind.

SAQ 2 (*Objectives 6 and 10*) In what main ways do PTH and Vitamin D act similarly with respect to blood calcium, and in what ways do they appear to act differently?

Sections 9.1 and 9.2.1

SAQ 3 (*Objective 10*)

(a) What is meant by the expression 'a push–pull system' in the context of calcium metabolism?

(b) Can you compare it with a similar mechanism in blood sugar regulation?

(c) Do you consider it differs in principle from all other homeostatic mechanisms you have met so far in Units 1–9 of this Course?

Section 9.2

SAQ 4 (*Objectives 7.1 and 7.2, 8 and 9*)

(a) What do you mean when you say that two hormones are acting antagonistically?

(b) Can the following pairs of hormones be said to be antagonists?
progesterone and oestrogen
adrenalin and insulin
glucagon and insulin
hydrocortisone and adrenalin

SAQ 5 (*Objective 7.2*) What effect do adrenalin and glucagon have on the level of blood sugar? Compare the similarities and dissimilarities of their modes of action and control.

Self-assessment Answers and Comments

SAQ 1

(a) The effect, predictably, is that the level of blood Ca is permanently very high.

(b) In spite of the high blood calcium, the continuous stimulation of the osteoclasts (and any other mechanism for the mobilization of 'non-exchangeable' bone) results in decalcification of the bones, which therefore become brittle and weak.

(c) This may not be immediately obvious to you. Look again at the answer to (b) above. What must happen to all the calcium mobilized from the bone?

As you would expect, the level of phosphate in the urine is high from the start; this is part of the normal effect of PTH. However, the sustained high blood level of calcium, derived from the bones, results in its excretion in the urine, because the kidney can no longer hold it back (see Unit 10). Thus, after a while, the urine shows high levels of both phosphate and calcium—in short, the bones are being dissolved and leaked out of the body.

SAQ 2

They both increase absorption of calcium by the gut, and the mobilization of non-exchangeable bone. Whereas PTH acts on the kidney to *increase* phosphate excretion and calcium retention, Vitamin D (at least in calcium deficiency) may cause phosphate retention by the kidney. This may have the effect of reducing the net loss of calcium from the bones.

SAQ 3

(a) It refers to a system where one hormone is concerned in the basic homeostatic response (in this case PTH, which has a direct negative feedback relationship with the calcium in the blood flowing through the parathyroid gland), but where another hormone has an opposite negative feedback relationship with the same substance (calcitonin and blood calcium). This may serve to prevent 'over-correction' by the first mechanism, or have some other function as yet undefined.

(b) It would seem to have a close parallel in the insulin-glucagon relationship in the blood sugar regulation of the mammal. In both cases, the stimulus for release is provided principally by changes in the level of the substance being regulated; in both cases, the stimulus is opposite (i.e. high blood glucose causes insulin release, which then depresses it; low blood sugar causes glucagon release, which then elevates it).

(c) This is really a matter of opinion, and in ours the answer is no. These are straightforward negative feedback responses which result in homeostasis; physiologically the two 'halves' of the push–pull may operate together and smooth out the response, wheras other similar homeostatic mechanisms may appear to operate separately in time (e.g. adrenalin and insulin), but it would seem doubtful if the mechanism is really different in principle.

SAQ 4

The main point of both parts (a) and (b) of this question is to emphasize the point that the phrase 'antagonistic' (or for that matter, 'synergistic') has no meaning in the context of hormone action unless it is precisely related to a particular event. Thus, if two hormones have opposite effects on a particular event in a particular place, it is meaningful, and sometimes useful, to describe them as acting antagonistically on that event in that place. Without such a close qualification, the term is useless, and raises all sorts of curious philosophical points. The phrase is usually used in a physiological rather than a biochemical context, describing an overall effect without any real implication as to fundamental processes.

(b) *Progesterone and oestrogen* are good examples. They act antagonistically on uterine muscle with regard to its resting muscle tone and sensitivity to the hormone oxytocin (see Home Experiment, Unit 8) for example. They show no generalized antagonism, and in fact often synergize some responses.

Adrenalin and insulin Yes, so far as the level of glucose in the blood is concerned, simply in that one tends to elevate it and the other to depress it. However, they act in quite different ways on quite different enzymes, so there is no direct interrelationship one way or the other.

Glucagon and insulin Yes, in so far as blood sugar levels are concerned. Exactly the same observations apply as to adrenalin and insulin.

Hydrocortisone and adrenalin This is an extreme case of the general point made in (a) above; the comparison is meaningless unless rigidly qualified. They act *synergistically* with respect to blood sugar levels, in that they both tend to elevate them, though by completely different pathways. They could be said to act *antagonistically* on the secretion of lactose by the mammary gland, however, in that hydrocortisone is important in providing the gland with glucose, whereas adrenalin, at least in moderately high physiological doses, reduces milk secretion and lactose production because it reduces the blood supply to the gland. (The mammary gland provides a very sensitive example of peripheral vasoconstriction, see Section 9.2.5 and Unit 5.)

We hope that you will use the phrase 'antagonistic action' with due care.

SAQ 5

Similarities in mode of action and control:

1 They both act to elevate blood sugar.

2 They do so by mobilizing liver glycogen→blood glucose.

3 They act on the phosphorylase-catalysed breakdown of glycogen to glucoses -1-P.

4 Cyclic-AMP mediates the effects of both on phosphorylase.

Dissimilarities in mode of action and control:

(1) Adrenalin stimulates the phosphorylase in muscle as well as liver cells, thus mobilizing muscle glycogen. Glucagon does not.

(2) Adrenalin has many other effects on the body, some of which will tend to increase the consumption of blood sugar (e.g. increase in heart and respiratory rate, heat production, etc.); glucagon does not.

(3) Glucagon release is triggered by a fall in the level of the sugar in blood circulating through the islets of Langerhans; this results directly in secretion by the α cells. Adrenalin release involves a nervous pathway from the hypothalamus, where the sugar-sensitive cells are located. Low blood sugar as such has no effect directly on the cells of the adrenal gland. Because of this difference, adrenalin release can take place even if the blood sugar is normal, with the result of elevating the sugar level above normal. Glucagon release appears to occur only in response to a low blood sugar.

(4) Weight for weight, glucagon is a more powerful agent for stimulating the phosphorylase system.

(5) Circulating adrenaline also inhibits insulin release; glucagon does not.

Hormones and Homeostasis: Osmoregulation and Excretion
Unit 10

Contents

Objectives

When you have read this text and the set reading you should be able to:

1   Define, recognize the best definitions of, or place in the correct context all the terms listed in Table A.

2   Describe or select correct descriptions of the physical problems presented by the major environments (marine, freshwater and terrestrial) to the animals living in them, especially with reference to osmoregulation and excretion.

3   Describe, or select correct descriptions of, the types of solutions to the osmotic and excretory problems posed by the environment, displayed by a hypothetical vertebrate or invertebrate, a mammal, a teleost or an arthropod.

4   Describe or select correct descriptions of two hormonal mechanisms involved in osmoregulation in vertebrates.

5   Account for osmoregulation in the mammal in terms of negative feedback systems.

6   Write a general account of the working of the mammalian kidney in 1 000 words.

7   Give at least two examples of the adaptation of an animal's excretory product to its mode of life and its environment.

The constancy of the internal environment is the necessary condition for independent life.

Claude Bernard (1813–1878)

Table A

List of Scientific Terms, Concepts and Principles used in Unit 10

Taken as prerequisites			Introduced in this Unit			
1 Assumed from general knowledge	**2** Introduced in a previous Unit	Unit No.	**3** Developed in this Unit or in its set book	Page No.	**4** Developed in a later Unit	Unit No.
	S22-		**In Unit**			
	osmosis, osmotic pressure	3	isosmotic cells	5		
	aldosterone	9	ionic regulation	6		
			osmoregulation	6		
	S100		excretion	8		
	elasmobranch	21	arginase	9		
	teleost	21	ornithine cycle	9		
	fish evolution	21	urea	9		
			uric acid	9		
			ultrafiltration	10		
			GFR	11		
			osmoreceptor	12		
			renin	12		
			angiotensin I and II	13		
			rectal gland	14		
			antennary glands	16		
			Malpighian tubule	17		
			contractile vacuole	19		
			In Moffat			
			nephron	3		
			glomerulus	3		
			proximal tubule	3		
			distal tubule	3		
			collecting duct	3		
			loop of Henle	3		
			renal cortex	3		
			renal medulla	3		
			renal papilla	3		
			osmolality	4		
			Bowman's capsule	6		
			hypo-osmotic	11		
			hyper-osmotic	11		
			anti-diuretic hormone	13		
			diuresis	13		

Study Guide

This Unit is something of a mixture of styles. Section 10.1 attempts to generalize about the osmotic problems posed by different environments, and why these affect different groups of animals in different ways. This sets the scene for the remainder of the Unit. Section 10.2 is a very brief one on nitrogenous excretion intended to explain the relationship between osmoregulation and excretion.

Section 10.3 on the mammalian kidney relies on the prescribed text *The Control of Water Balance by the Kidney* by D. B. Moffat (1971) Oxford University Press, (20p). It will be referred to as Moffat.

Section 10.3.1 is a short commentary on this booklet which is essential reading unless you are fully conversant with the physiology of the mammalian kidney. The questions which follow are also important because they emphasize the two aspects of the functioning of the nephron, the 'mechanical' nature of glomerular function, and the flexible nature of control of the distal tubular function.

Section 10.3.2 briefly described the role of hormones in the control of osmo-regulatory action by the kidney, and you should make mental comparisons between these examples of hormone action and those in Units 8 and 9.

Sections 10.4 and 10.5 consist of a very brief look at some of the solutions to the problems raised in 10.1, shown by other vertebrates and some invertebrates.

10.0 Introduction

In Unit 9 we looked at the involvement of various hormones in two homeostatic processes: the maintenance of constant levels of calcium and glucose in the blood. In the latter case we also considered how controlled variation of the level could be achieved. We confined our attention mainly to mammals because detailed knowledge of these mechanisms only exists for mammals; the equivalent work has yet to be done for other species. We confined our attention to these mechanisms partly because the substances being regulated are important physiologically, but also because they provide clear illustrations of the ways in which hormones may control homeostatic systems.

Just as fundamental to the organism as the regulation of calcium and glucose, however, is the regulation of the level of the nitrogenous waste products of protein metabolism in and around the cells, and also the ionic and osmotic concentrations of the fluids inside and outside the cell. There are severe limitations to the environmental changes that most animal cells can tolerate; therefore, if the environment in which the whole animal lives is widely different from the environment in which its individual cells can live, the animal must surround its cells with an artificial environment of the required standard. This is patently true with regard to the environmental levels of salts and osmotic concentration. You may recall that in Unit 6 we referred to the immediate and unfortunate effects of introducing freshwater (via the lungs) into the bloodstream, with a consequent lowering of its osmotic pressure. With regard to the nitrogenous waste which arises from the deamination of the amino acids in the course of metabolism, the necessity is to keep the level within the cell *below* certain limits rather than at a particular level; however, the problems of removal of nitrogenous wastes from metabolising cells (which is *excretion*) and the regulation of the ionic and osmotic concentrations often overlap.

Although osmoregulation and excretion have been studied over a much greater range of species than have either calcium or blood-sugar regulation, the part played by hormones in the control of the mechanisms is not known in such detail. For this reason, this Unit should give you a better *comparative* view of the physiology of homeostatic mechanisms than Unit 9, but perhaps a less explicit account of the ways in which hormones co-ordinate the mechanisms.

10.1 The Need to Regulate the Ionic and Osmotic Concentration of the Tissues

Life appears to have evolved initially in the sea (S100,* Unit 21), and the entire evolutionary history of the majority of the invertebrates now living there seems to have been spent in this same environment. It is therefore not surprising to find that their enzyme systems, and intra-cellular metabolism generally, have evolved in such a way that they function at an osmotic concentration virtually identical to that of sea water. Where reliable measurements have been made, the osmotic concentration of the intracellular contents (or cell 'sap') is identical to or within 2 per cent of, the osmotic concentration of sea water. Thus, no physiological work need be done to preserve the osmotic integrity of these cells, and there will be no large net movement of water due to osmosis, either into or out of the cells.

isosmotic cells

However, this is not to say that the concentrations of individual ions will be the same inside the cells and in the surrounding sea—frequently they are not. For one thing, much of the osmotic pressure of the cell sap is due to the colloids in it (see Unit 6, Section 6.1.1), notably the free amino acids. These will be virtually absent in the surrounding sea, yet if the total osmotic pressures of both the cell sap and the sea are the same, obviously the concentration of dissolved salts must be lower inside the cell. Furthermore, even the relative proportions of different ions may vary inside and outside the cell.

---

* *The Open University (1971) S100* Science: A Foundation Course, *The Open University Press.*

5

For example, the sap of most cells, particularly nerve and muscle cells, has a higher concentration of potassium ions and a lower concentration of sodium ions than the fluid outside them. The maintenance of this difference involves the cell in the expenditure of energy. Thus, even where osmotic work is not being performed, ionic pumping may well occur.

ionic pumping

Where the animal is uni-cellular, such work will be performed at the cell membrane. In the case of a metazoan animal whose cells are bathed in a body fluid, it is clearly possible that the body fluid will have the same proportions of ions as sea water, in which case the work will be done at each individual cell membrane just as if each was a unicell. On the other hand, some or all of this work may be done by specialized cells, forming the boundary between the sea and the body fluid; in this case, the body fluid may represent a half-way stage—spreading the load, so to speak—or it may be identical with the cell sap. In cases such as the Na/K ratio in 'excitable' cells (for example, nerve and muscle cells) it is essential that there shall be differences in the concentrations of these ions across the cell membranes—otherwise the conduction of nerve impulses and the contraction of muscle cells cannot take place. It is not surprising therefore to see (Table 1) that the proportions of sodium and potassium are very similar in the sea water and the plasma of an active marine crustacean, the shore-crab *Carcinus*; this is a case where the work is being done at each cell membrane. However, active fast-moving marine crustaceans maintain a lower concentration of magnesium ions throughout the body than is found in the surrounding sea water; thus the circulating plasma of *Carcinus* has a lower concentration than sea water (Table 1), which involves work at the plasma/sea water boundary, probably at the gills in fact.

Table I Comparison of the concentrations of three ions in sea water and two species of crustacean, expressed as relative concentrations where the chloride concentration is 100.

	Na	K	Mg	Cl
Sea water	55·5	2·01	6·69	100
Carcinus (shore-crab)	62·0	2·43	2·4	100
Lithodes (stone-crab)	58·0	2·56	6·7	100

(It has been suggested that the magnesium ion lowers the maximum speed at which the nerves and muscles can operate; the much more sluggish stone-crab *Lithodes* does not expend energy maintaining a difference.)

10.1.1 Regulation in a dilute medium

Ionic regulation may occur even where osmoregulation is unnecessary. However, when a marine invertebrate group begins to colonize a totally new medium, such as brackish estuarine waters or even freshwater, much more profound difficulties have to be overcome. When the animal moves into water with a lower osmotic pressure than sea water, water will tend to be drawn into the plasma, and then into the cells, by osmosis. This tendency has to be counteracted; unlike plant cells, animal cells have no rigid wall which enables them to develop a high hydrostatic (turgor) pressure to balance the osmotic pressure differences. Under these circumstances animal cells will swell and burst. If this is to be avoided, the osmotic pressure of the body fluids must be kept close to that of the cell sap.

osmotic uptake

QUESTION If a marine metazoan species attempts to colonize freshwater, what general categories of physiological action are open to it to prevent a fatal difference developing between the osmotic pressure of its plasma and that of its cells?

ANSWER In theory it could: (a) allow the plasma to become dilute, but develop a system in which each cell pumped out surplus water; (b) develop a body surface that was completely impermeable to water; (c) develop cell sap with a very low osmotic pressure; (d) keep the plasma fairly concentrated by pumping out all of the surplus water as it comes in; or (e) do all of these to some extent.

In practice, it seems that (e) is the usual state of affairs, but different species emphasize one or more of the above alternatives.

The majority of fresh- (or brackish-) water metazoans do not depend primarily on (a), possibly because a large proportion of both the anatomy and energy expenditure of each cell would be involved in osmoregulation. This is likely to be energetically wasteful, and in species with highly specialized cells it may also be anatomically undesirable, interfering with the specialized function. Nevertheless, some animals with a simpler tissue organization do appear to osmoregulate cell by cell, for example the freshwater cnidarians such as *Hydra* [*IS* 1]. It is far from clear how these animals avoid taking large amounts of water into their cells and retaining it; there is no good evidence that their cells are particularly waterproof, and if they were, it would be expected to lead to their being oxygen-proof as well, as we discussed in Unit 6. The cell sap, although more dilute than that of many freshwater animals, exerts a pressure of some 5mOsm/kg (see Moffat, p. 4 for an explanation of *osmolality* and its units) and so it will undoubtedly tend to draw water into the cells. Yet the individual cells show no evidence of any obvious pumping mechanism such as may be seen in many of the freshwater unicells (Section 10.5.2), so the energetics of osmoregulation in these animals remains a fascinating enigma.

[IS 1 = Cnidaria A and B]

The difficulty for our hypothetical animal in developing a surface totally impermeable to water—solution (b)—is that touched on above and in Unit 6, Section 6.1, namely that all the biological membranes so far investigated and found to be impervious to water are also impervious to dissolved oxygen. Thus, where a surface must allow the passage of oxygen sufficiently rapidly to meet the metabolic need, it seems it will also allow the inward diffusion of water. The only escape route for the animal from this dilemma will be to breathe oxygen from the air, rather than oxygen dissolved in the water; if it can do this it may be able to make all the surfaces in contact with the water impermeable. (See Unit 6, Section 6.3.4, Aquatic respiration by insects.)

The difficulties associated with solution (c), abandoning the ancestral composition of the cells, are insuperable. In the terms used in Unit 3, the water potential of the cell cytoplasm is bound to be lower than that of freshwater. The enzyme systems, common to all living systems on this planet, will not function in the absence of dissolved ions (nor is the integrity of the cell membrane retained in their absence) and there are bound to be colloids in the cell. Thus, although it is possible for species (and individuals) to adapt to some extent, there will always be a considerable difference in the osmotic pressure exerted by the cell contents and that of freshwater.

Solution (d) is one adopted by many species, often in conjunction with some of the others. Thus, the osmotic concentration of the plasma is prevented from falling too low by pumping out the surplus water which enters through the gills and elsewhere. However, the plasma may not be as concentrated as sea water indicating that the cells are able to tolerate lower osmotic pressures than in marine forms; elements of solutions (a) and (c) may be present here. Frequently also the entire body surface except the gills is made impermeable (b), reducing the inflow of water to the minimum. This system (d) will, of course, require energy to maintain itself; the water pump may be a hydrostatic one, as in vertebrates and some crustaceans (Section 10.5), where the energy is derived from the heart; or it may be an electrochemical device of some kind (Section 10.5.1) possibly of the kind discussed in Unit 3 in plant phloem. In any event, to maintain such a difference between the plasma and the environment will require work.

10.1.2   Regulation in a terrestrial environment

The move from a seawater environment to a freshwater one is, of course, not the only move posing osmotic problems. The colonization of land presents its own problems, and these are essentially similar whether the change is from a freshwater or a marine environment. Basically, the osmotic problems of terrestrial organisms stem from loss of water due to evaporation. How acute the problem of evaporative loss is will depend on various factors, notably the actual habitat of the particular species. Thus, there is a difference of degree in the osmotic problems of an animal living in the North African desert and one living under a wet log in a Dorset wood, but only rarely is there a difference in kind. (There *are* examples

evaporation

7

of quite different problems; for example the earthworm, whilst in its normal habitat in the soil, tends to take up soil water by osmosis and thus it shares some of the problems of an animal in freshwater; however, when it is on the surface, evaporative loss of water becomes a major hazard.)

If a terrestrial animal protects itself against the loss of water by evaporation by making its body surface impermeable to water, it will once again encounter the respiratory problems mentioned above. So the respiratory surfaces will be moist (Unit 6) and a site of water loss. Furthermore, a terrestrial animal may require water to dispose of its nitrogenous waste (Section 10.2) which will place a further load on the water supply.

The loss of water will, of course, tend to raise the osmotic levels of the plasma which, among other effects, will withdraw water from the cells—a process that may prove rapidly fatal. The only way a terrestrial animal can make good this water loss is through the gut—making use of water derived from the food or by actually drinking water. Thus, water regulation in terrestrial animals is based on an essentially conservative system, often supported by particular behaviour patterns designed to minimize water loss.

10.1.3 Marine vertebrates

There is another environmental osmotic problem which has to be faced by many vertebrates, and that is the *recolonization* of the sea. The early vertebrate history has been an entirely estuarine and freshwater one; thus the basic physiology of vertebrates has evolved round a system for ridding the body of surplus water (Section 10.4). In addition to the development of an excretory organ (the kidney) highly adapted to this purpose, the process of dilution of the plasma (and a corresponding drop in the osmotic pressure of the intracellular contents) which reduces the osmotic intake of water, has also occurred. Thus the plasma of a freshwater fish has an osmotic pressure only about one-third that of sea water. In the Devonian era, some 350 million years ago, fish began to colonize the sea, the first vertebrates to do so. Unlike the native inhabitants, the fish were faced with an acute water shortage, as water must have been drawn from the plasma across the gills by the higher osmotic pressure exerted by the sea water. The ways in which this problem is solved by the living descendants of the original colonists, and by other marine vertebrates, is discussed later in this Unit; the point to remember at the moment is that this problem is faced by very few (if any) animals other than the vertebrates, but it applies to all vertebrates re-colonizing the sea.

marine vertebrates

10.2 Nitrogenous Excretion

It may not be altogether clear to you at this point why we are considering excretion at the same time as osmoregulation, particularly in a Unit concerned with homeostasis and hormones. Except in a very few special cases (Section 10.4) excretory systems do not maintain nitrogenous waste materials at a particular level, but maintain them *below* a particular level—a rather different situation to the ones we have looked at as homeostasis previously. Furthermore, this regulation is not directly controlled by hormones. The reason we consider osmoregulation and excretion together, however, is because in many animals they are closely interlinked in terms of actual physiological function. In terrestrial animals in particular, it is not possible to consider osmoregulation separately from excretion.

The breakdown of amino acids occurs continually in almost all the animals whose metabolism has been studied, even in starvation. If the animal is on a high protein diet, much of its energy will be derived from protein and the amount of amino-acid breakdown will be correspondingly higher. An amino acid must be de-aminated—i.e. the terminal NH_2 group removed—before the carbon skeleton can be used as a fuel. The result of this breakdown is the production of ammonia, NH_3

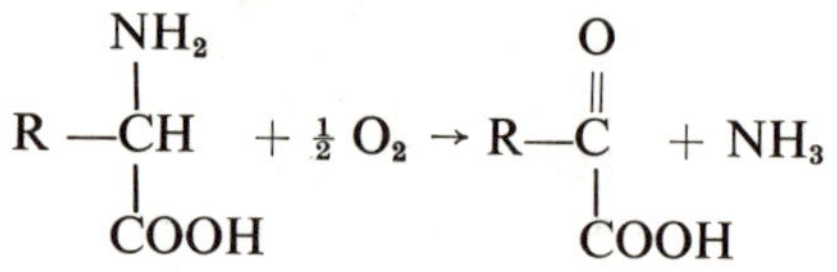

$$R-\underset{\underset{COOH}{|}}{\overset{\overset{NH_2}{|}}{CH}} + \tfrac{1}{2}O_2 \rightarrow R-\underset{\underset{COOH}{|}}{\overset{\overset{O}{\|}}{C}} + NH_3$$

Figure 1 De-amination of an amino acid.

8

Unfortunately, ammonia is highly toxic, so it must be disposed of rapidly as it is formed, without the level in the body fluids rising too high. An aquatic animal with a large permeable area in contact with the water can lose its ammonia fast enough by simple diffusion; the concentration gradient of ammonia will be steep even when the internal level is still quite low, because under normal circumstances the level of ammonia in the medium is negligible. Thus, all aquatic animals which breathe dissolved oxygen, either through gills or the body wall (which in unicells is the cell membrane), are able to dispose of much of their nitrogenous waste as ammonia, by allowing it to diffuse out into the surrounding medium. In many cases, almost all the waste nitrogen is lost this way, in others it may be about 90 per cent. In teleost fish, some 90 per cent diffuses out through the gills, though not all as ammonia.

However, in animals where water is not available in unlimited quantities and in close association with the blood, this system will not work. For example, air-breathing animals cannot dispose of NH_3 in this way; the concentration of dissolved ammonia in the blood would have to be enormous before it began to come out of solution into the air, in any quantity—the animal would be dead long before this happened.* Animals unable to get rid of ammonia by diffusion possess enzyme systems which enable them to combine it with other substances to form less harmful compounds. (Even in cases where water *is* available this may happen—for example, many fish, particularly marine teleosts, manufacture** a substance called trimethylamine oxide, which is largely responsible for the 'fishy' smell of fish. For quite different reasons, dealt with later in the Unit, the cartilaginous (Elasmobranch) fish combine their ammonia with carbon dioxide to produce *urea*.)

Many vertebrates produce urea and, those which do so, possess the enzyme *arginase*. The urea is produced by the so-called *ornithine cycle* (Fig. 2), discovered by Krebs in 1932, before his other and more celebrated cycle. Urea is relatively non-toxic and very soluble. It is therefore very suitable for excretion by the kidney, provided a reasonable amount of water is available. Adult amphibia produce some urea, although the eggs and young aquatic larvae produce ammonia. Animals with shelled eggs that develop on land have some special problems in this respect.

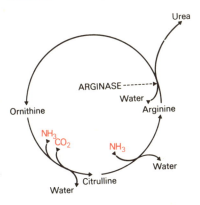

ammonia

Figure 2 The ornithine cycle. Urea is synthesized from ammonia and carbon dioxide.

urea

ornithine cycle

Can you think what they are?

Thus a different excretory product would seem to be called for.

What characteristics would seem desirable in the excretory product of an embryo in a shelled egg?

1 Ammonia will not be suitable as the major excretory product because the eggs are not surrounded by water.
2 Urea is very soluble but, as it cannot escape, it will accumulate in the egg and exert a very high osmotic pressure which may damage the embryo.

1 It should be non-toxic.
2 It should not exert a high osmotic pressure when its concentration in the egg rises.

The substance produced by most animals that lay their eggs on dry land is in fact uric acid, which has both the properties suggested. It does not exert a high osmotic pressure because it is rather insoluble, and as the concentration rises it crystallizes out of solution and becomes biologically inert. Thus, the hatching embryo can merely leave sludge of uric acid crystals behind it in the shell.

Uric acid (Fig. 3) is the main excretory product of insects, terrestrial gastropod molluscs, reptiles (except some aquatic ones) and birds. From what has been said, it will be apparent that in animals where the nitrogen is lost by diffusion there will be little direct connection between the processes of excretion and osmoregulation. This is true of the vertebrates, and teleost fish show no such connection (elasmobranchs are a special case, as they produce urea). Thus, the

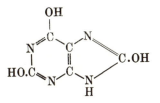

Figure 3 Uric acid.

---

* *Some woodlice appear to be an exception to this generalization.*

** *There is considerable doubt as to whether the majority of the trimethylamine oxide is endogenous or whether it is eaten with the food.*

vertebrate kidney functions in its earlier forms as an osmoregulatory device, a water pump, not as an organ of excretion. This latter function is taken on by the vertebrate kidney only in terrestrial forms (or those which are secondarily aquatic).

10.3 The Mammalian Kidney

In this Section, we consider the mechanisms for achieving osmotic homeostasis in mammals. We begin with mammals rather than other animals, because much more is known about the control of osmoregulation in mammals than in any other group of animals.

Now READ the booklet *The control of water balance by the kidney* by D. B. Moffat, which comprises the set reading for this Unit. The anatomy and basic working of the mammalian kidney are clearly described, though at a fairly elementary level. We offer you a brief commentary and some questions to help you with it, but we *assume* that you have read it before you continue with this Section, and for this reason we carry straight on to elaborate on the control mechanisms.

10.3.1 The set text: Moffat

Up to p. 8, the text is mainly a descriptive account of the functional anatomy of the mammal kidney. You should be able to recall what is meant by the words in italics (they are listed in Table A, p. 3). Although you should appreciate how the structure of the glomerulus enables it to act as a filter, it is not worth committing the names of the structures of the epithelium (podocytes, pedicels etc.) to memory. You will notice that, although we regarded the basement membranes of epithelia as rather inert structures in the histology text (Home Experiment associated with Unit 4), in this case the membrane is playing a very important functional role. Incidentally, our photomicrograph (filmstrip 1, frame Fs1.1) of the glomerulus is very much better than Figure 3b in the text—so look at FS 1.1 again!

mammal kidney

glomerulus

The process by which the glomerular filtrate is produced (filtration under pressure) is generally known as *ultrafiltration*.

ultrafiltration

On p. 11, the statement is made that 'only birds and mammals are able to produce a concentrated urine'. This may be misleading—the Open University authors do not know of evidence of bird urine containing a solution of salts more concentrated than the blood, nor of urine with a higher overall osmotic pressure than the blood.

You are already familiar with countercurrent systems from Unit 6, Appendix 2, where the example quoted for a 'hairpin' system was the heat exchanger in the heron's leg. In theory, the osmotic gradients, once set up, could be maintained indefinitely by the arrangement of the tubules, without any further work being necessary. In practice, of course, sodium pumping will be required because (a) the system is not physically perfect and (b) because the fluid in the papilla may be diluted by filtrate drawn in from the collecting ducts.

countercurrent

At the bottom of p. 13, the sentence beginning 'The permeability of the distal tubule . . .' and running over on to p. 14 may confuse you. The changes in the distal tubule which cause increased sodium and water reabsorption do not cause 'increased concentration of the fluid' in the sense that they make it hyperosmotic to the blood. If ADH is secreted, the fluid in the distal tubule will merely tend to *equilibrate* osmotically with the blood (remember it emerges from the ascending loop slightly *hyposmotic*), and if sodium is pumped back into the blood at the same time it will carry with it additional water, but *isosmotically*. Thus, the volume of filtrate in the distal tube may be reduced dramatically, but it is not concentrated relative to the blood.

distal tubule

If you want to see the appearance of the cells of the tubules in the region of the distal tubule and small collecting ducts (i.e. at the top right of the diagram on p. 3) you should examine the histology filmstrip 1, frame Fs 1.6.

If you have already viewed the TV programme of Unit 10, the electron micrograph in Figure 11b should look rather familiar. It bears marked similarities to the one we showed you of the base of an epithelial cell from the lining of the tubes of the 'unknown organ'.

You should attempt the questions below before continuing with the Main Text.

QUESTION If we accept the figure of 70–75 mmHg as being the pressure of the blood in the glomerular capillaries (p. 8) and subtract 2–3 mmHg for the resistance offered by the endothelium of the capillaries and the epithelium of the capsule, what do you think the *net filtration pressure* will be? That is to say, what will be the pressure actually available to force liquid into the tubule (and thus the hydrostatic pressure of the filtrate in the glomerular end of the proximal tubule)?

ANSWER If you said 70–75 mm minus 3 mm, therefore giving a net filtration pressure of around 67–72 mmHg you were being forgetful: Moffat explains that the longer molecules do not cross the membranes. You will recall that when we considered filtration into the alveolus of the lung (Unit 6, Section 6.1.1, p. 8) we said that the plasma proteins and other colloids exerted an osmotic pressure (the colloid osmotic pressure) which amounted to about 25 mmHg in mammals. This pressure will be exerted in the opposite direction to the hydrostatic pressure—tending to pull water back into the capillary. Thus, a more accurate calculation of the net filtration pressure would be 70 (or 75)—3—25 = 42. In this context, it is interesting to note the very large difference in the pressure of the blood in lung capillaries (28 mmHg) and glomerular ones (70–75 mmHg).

net filtration pressure

QUESTION 2 If you restricted the renal artery with a clamp so that the blood pressure in the kidney fell to about 40 mmHg, what do you think would happen to the production of urine?

ANSWER 2 It would cease, because the glomerular filtration rate (GFR) (the rate at which filtrate emerges from the glomerulus, usually measured in cm³/min) would fall to zero when the hydrostatic pressure available for ultrafiltration fell to less than the sum of the colloid osmotic pressure and the glomerular resistance.

GFR

QUESTION 3 Various drugs may affect the diameter of the afferent or efferent arterioles of the glomerulus. For example, caffeine causes vasodilation of the afferent arteriole, and adrenalin causes vasoconstriction of the efferent arteriole. What effect do you think the administration of (a) caffeine and (b) adrenalin will have on the GFR—the amount of filtrate produced per minute?

ANSWER 3 (a) Vasodilation of the *afferent* arteriole will increase the blood pressure in the glomerulus and thus increase GFR. (This usually leads to increased urine production—hence the well-known effect of coffee.)
(b) Vasoconstriction of the *efferent* arteriole will similarly lead to increased glomerular pressure and GFR.

QUESTION 4 Question 3 made it clear that it would have been quite possible for mammals to have evolved a system to control the rate of urine production (and thus water loss) by simply varying the GFR. When the animal was short of water, the GFR could be reduced by vasoconstriction of the afferent arteriole, when it was water-loaded the glomerular pressure could be raised. Nevertheless, Moffat makes it quite clear (p. 9) that the normal variation in urine production (between 0·3 cm³ and 20 cm³ per min in man) is achieved by different treatments of only 10 or 15 per cent of the filtrate after it reaches the distal tubule.
Can you think of any advantages to the species in having adopted the latter rather than the former system?

ANSWER 4 85–90 per cent of the filtrate is reabsorbed by the proximal tubule ('obligatory reabsorption'); thus, in order to change the excretion of urine from the body by a few cm³ per minute, very large changes would have to occur in the amount of glomerular filtrate formed, and thus of blood filtered. For example, reducing the urine flow from 10 cm³/min to 1 cm³/min might require the amount of glomerular filtrate formed to be reduced from 125 cm³/min to 12·5. This would mean that in times of anti-diuresis the blood would scarcely be cleared of urea and other waste products at all.

QUESTION 5 The molecular weight of haemoglobin (67 000) represents the borderline size of molecule which is filtered out by the glomerulus. Why does haemoglobin not normally appear in the blood?

ANSWER 5 Because the haemoglobin is contained in red blood cells. If these are ruptured in large numbers, haemoglobin does appear in the urine and, what is more, it may block the glomerular 'sieve'. This can happen in infections by haemolytic bacteria, including some streptococci.

10.3.2 Control of water excretion by the mammalian kidney

It can be shown that a change of 1 per cent in the osmotic pressure of a mammal may result in a reduction in urine flow of up to 90 per cent. As suggested in Moffat, much of this change is due to the action of a polypeptide hormone secreted by the nervous tissue of the *posterior* lobe of pituitary gland. Precursors of this hormone are secreted by nerves in the hypothalamus, and travel down the nerve axons into the posterior lobe. This hormone, anti-diuretic hormone (ADH), is also known as *vasopressin*.

vasopressin (ADH)

The mechanism was first isolated by Verney in 1947. He was trying to locate the receptors responsible for causing anti-diuresis by perfusing hypertonic saline solutions into experimental animals. He discovered that a small quantity of hypertonic saline solution introduced into the carotid artery would induce anti-diuresis—reduction in urine flow—even though the general blood osmotic pressure did not justify this. The same amount of saline injected elsewhere did not have this effect. Thus it appeared that the receptors were in the brain. It also appeared that they were *osmoreceptors* not receptors sensitive to salt levels, as non-saline solutions of comparable osmolality had the same effect. These receptors are now known to be located in the hypothalamus, close to a region known as the supra-optic nucleus.

osmoreceptors

Thus, there is a negative feedback system, in which blood osmotic pressure is monitored by receptors; if the osmotic pressure rises, ADH release is stimulated and the urine flow is reduced—in man to as little as 0·1–0·3 cm³/min (derived from an original filtrate of 125 cm³/min.).

However, these very low levels of urine flow can only be achieved if the blood level of urea is not high. Urea exerts a high osmotic pressure, and thus if the amount of protein in the diet is high, then the urea will carry considerable quantities of water out with it. As suggested in Moffat, the degree to which the osmotic pressure of the urine may be raised depends on the length of the loops of Henle. In some desert rats with very long loops, provided the diet is a low-protein one, the animals can live on metabolic water (that derived from the oxidation of the foodstuffs) alone.

There are, of course, occasions when the body is overloaded with water and short of salt. In this case, ADH secretion will cease (no stimulation of the osmo-receptors) and the maximum effort will be made to recover Na ions from the distal tubule. This latter procedure is stimulated by the secretion of the mineralo-corticoid *aldosterone* (see Unit 9) from the adrenal cortex. This acts partly by accelerating the Na pumps in the distal tubule. If aldosterone secretion is accompanied by ADH secretion, then water follows the sodium isosmotically out of the tubule and into the blood. If ADH is absent, the distal tubule seems to be fairly waterproof, and Na is pumped out leaving the water behind—giving a large flow of dilute filtrate into the collecting duct; this will then pass down the collecting duct relatively unchanged.

aldosterone

One stimulus for the release of aldosterone is a change in the proportion of Na and K in the plasma circulating through the adrenal gland. Thus, if Na falls relative to K, aldosterone is released and the Na pumps in the tubule exchange Na in the filtrate for K in the plasma.

However, there is another very elegant feedback relationship between the kidney and aldosterone release. If there is serious haemorrhage, or the blood pressure falls for any other reason, a group of cells situated around the afferent and efferent glomerular arterioles are stimulated to release a hormone *renin*. This circulates in the plasma and acts on a substance always present called angio-

renin

12

tensin I to convert it into a highly active form called angiotensin II. This substance has two main effects: one is to raise blood pressure (and thus restore the GFR, which will have declined as a result in the drop in pressure) by increasing cardiac output and peripheral resistance; the other is to stimulate aldosterone release and thus Na retention by the body. This latter step is important if the body fluid volume is to be maintained.

angiotensin I and II

Thus we have a system where the kidney is acting as a homeostat on blood pressure to maintain its own GFR, in addition to the effect on electrolyte balance.

We have given an immensely simplified version of renal function here. Not only have we skated over the method of action of aldosterone and ADH, but we have not considered the action of parathyroid hormone on Ca and PO_4, or the factors controlling acid/base regulation (to name just two systems you know of). However, we hope it has served to explain the general principles.

10.4   Comparative Kidney Function in Vertebrates

Fish

Fish evolved in freshwater; and modern freshwater fish have blood which is about one-third the osmolality of sea water—about 300 mOsm/l compared to about 940 mOsm/l. They have a skin which is impermeable, and they can also take up ions from the medium via special cells in the gills. Water enters the body across the gills by osmosis; their kidneys function much in the same way as did their ancestors 400 million years ago—they act as a water pump, but recover most of the salts from the filtrate. They produce a flow of urine equal to 8 or 9 per cent of their body weight per day, but it has only about 1/50 of the plasma concentration of salt. Thus they are taking at least three of the courses open to an animal osmoregulating in freshwater. Marine teleost fish, as mentioned earlier, have the opposite problem: their blood has about a half the osmolality of sea water. Thus, they do not filter with the kidney; in some cases this shutdown is physiological, in others it is due to anatomical changes—the glomeruli have actually been lost from the kidney (e.g. the angler fish, *Lophius*). In some groups, the glomeruli are still present in small numbers or in the larvae only. Thus we are witnessing an evolutionary process whereby teleosts are becoming fully adapted to a marine environment. Teleost fish with aglomerular kidneys produce a very small quantity of hypotonic urine by active secretion from the tubules. However, reducing the urine flow does not solve the problem of lost water (and extra salt acquired by inward diffusion), it only mitigates it. Thus, marine fish must drink sea water, absorb it and most of its salts through the gut, and then pump out surplus salts across the gills back into the sea—a process requiring much energy.

marine teleosts

Migratory teleosts, such as the trout, salmon and eel have to be able to adapt to both sets of conditions. The trout and salmon are primarily freshwater fish—they lay their eggs in freshwater—and they function as perfectly normal freshwater fish whilst in rivers and lakes. When they migrate to the sea they have to stop the urine flow (they reduce it by about 99 per cent) and begin to drink sea water. When they first enter the sea, they reduce the urine flow by reducing the GFR, but when they are fully adapted, in about three days, the GFR rises again, but the water is reabsorbed. There is evidence that posterior lobe hormones are involved in this. The plasma osmolality is allowed to rise from one-third to one-half that of sea water. The kidney cannot produce a urine more concentrated than the blood, as it has no loops of Henle, so it is of no positive value for osmoregulation in the sea. Several groups of fish left the rivers for the sea as long ago as the Devonian, some 75 million years before the ancestors of the teleosts did so (S100, Unit 21). These fish, including the Elasmobranchs and the Crossopterygians, evolved a mechanism for osmoregulation which is more economical than that of the marine teleosts. Their kidney is designed to retain 80–90 per cent of the urea in the blood, and their tissues produce urea rather than ammonia or trimethylamine oxide. Thus the level of urea in the blood is allowed to rise until the osmolality of the plasma is the same as that of the surrounding sea water. Thus, there is no net water loss by osmosis. The same process is shown by the crab-eating frog, *Rana cancrivora*, which lives in

Elasmobranchs

13

estuaries and brackish lagoons in S.E. Asia. (An amphibian, with its permeable skin, would normally be expected to shrivel and die rapidly in sea water.)

However, although the urea in the blood of elasmobranchs means they do not lose water, they will gain salt, because their blood has a salinity about half that of sea water (Fig. 4), so that diffusion will take place down the Na concentration gradient from the sea water. They cope with this by having a special salt-secretory gland (the rectal gland) which produces a secretion with a higher salt concentration even than sea water. (It is only isosmotic with the plasma, but this is irrelevant, as the value to the animal is in the removal of surplus salt.)

rectal gland

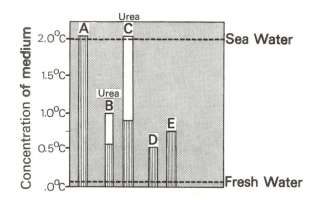

Figure 4   *A comparison of the concentration of the blood of various fishes.*

A *Myxine*, B *Pristis*, C shark, D freshwater teleost, E marine teleost

reptiles and birds

The reptiles and birds operate a water-conservative excretory system (except for some freshwater aquatic reptiles such as the crocodile) even though their loops of Henle are poorly developed. They achieve this by two means. First, the excretory product is uric acid, which is insoluble—thus it can be precipitated out in the kidney, emerging rather like toothpaste, and taking very little water with it. Second, marine species have, in addition, special salt secretory glands, not unlike those of the elasmobranchs; these operate on a countercurrent principle with the blood, and involve large 'batteries' of Na pumps. These can produce a fluid hypertonic to sea water.

Some birds, e.g. the chicken, recover some of the water necessary to carry the uric acid out of the kidney, and they do it by a rather surprising manoeuvre. When the urine leaves the ureters and enters the cloaca (the common opening of the gut, ureters and genital tract), it is drawn up into the gut by peristalsis and carried to a region of the hind gut where water absorption takes place. The uric acid crystals then pass out with the faeces.

We can perhaps best summarize the vertebrate situation in the following two figures.

Figure 4 shows the osmolality of the blood of various fishes in fresh and sea water. Column A shows the blood concentration of the hagfish (*Myxine*), an animal we have not mentioned. It is a cyclostome, rather similar to the lamprey you saw in the TV programme of Unit 8, but it feeds on marine invertebrates. It is marine, and a descendant of the ancient armoured jawless fish, the earliest vertebrates. Little is known of its history, but its blood is isosmotic with sea water, like a marine invertebrate.

Column C shows the blood of an elasmobranch, such as a shark or dogfish, in sea water, and column B, an elasmobranch in freshwater—the freshwater sawfish, *Pristis*. The high osmolality of the plasma with urea causes a very large urine flow in freshwater, and this leaches out a proportion of the urea. If the animal is moved to sea water, the urea level rises to a normal elasmobranch level. Columns D and E show the blood of a freshwater and a marine teleost respectively.

Figure 5 is a diagrammatic representation of the nephrons in the kidneys of various vertebrates.

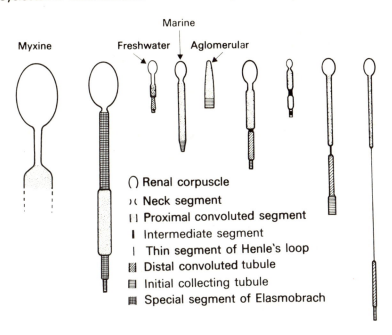

Figure 5   *Diagrammatic comparison of various vertebrate nephrons.*

How might the kidney of a marine teleost produce a small flow of hypo-osmotic urine?

If Na is actively secreted into the proximal tubule, water will follow isosmotically. If some of the Na is then reabsorbed in the distal tubule, the urine will be hypotonic.

10.5   Invertebrate Osmoregulatory Patterns

A most interesting illustration of the ways in which a group of animals may adapt to the different environments is provided by the *crustaceans* [*IS 1*]. They are a primarily marine group, but they have very successfully colonized freshwater and, rather less successfully, the land.

Some crustacean species are quite unable to osmoregulate, so if the water becomes more or less concentrated than normal sea water, the blood concentration follows. An example of this is the spider-crab, *Maia* (Fig. 6). Others, like the shore-crab *Carcinus* can reduce the permeability of the gills when in brackish water and also pick up Na from the water to make good the loss in the urine, which is isosmotic with the blood. *Carcinus* can also tolerate a lowered plasma osmolality, and adjust the concentration of the cell sap; this is partly achieved by a marked drop in the intracellular concentration of amino acids.

[IS 1 = Arthropoda A and B, Arthropoda C]

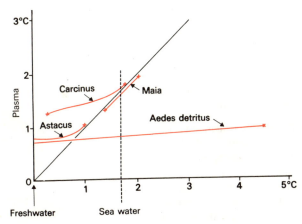

Figure 6   *Effect of the osmotic pressure of the medium on the body fluids of four arthropods.*

The main excretory organs of the malacostracan crustaceans are paired antennary glands. These secrete urine into a bladder via a tubule. The urine is isosmotic with the blood in marine forms, and the evidence is that it is formed by a process of ultra-filtration. In freshwater forms, the tubule between the gland and the bladder is long and coiled, and plays an important part in recovering salt from the urine, which emerges hypo-osmotic (Fig. 7a and b). A crustacean which can live permanently in fresh water is the crayfish *Astacus*. The permeability of the body is low compared to marine crustaceans, i.e. 370 M/kg of Na escapes per hour compared to between 1 000 and 2 000 M/kg/hr in marine forms. Salts are secreted inwards by the gills to compensate, and a dilute urine is produced by the antennary glands. It is quite interesting to compare its osmotic performance with that of the trout in fresh water, as is done in Table 1.

Table 1

	Urine flow	Urine Concn.	Plasma Concn.
Crayfish	3·4 cm³/Kg/hr	6 mM/l Na	203 mM/l Na
Trout	3·6 cm³/Kg/hr	2–11 mM/l Na	290 mM/l Na

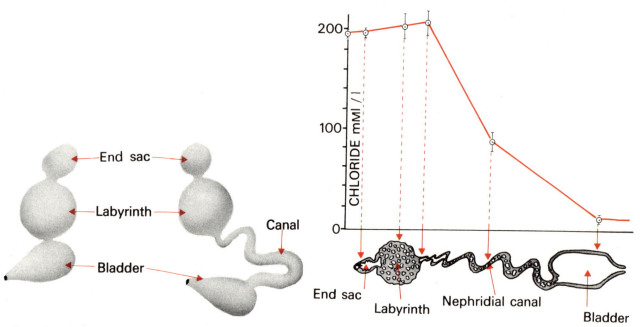

Figure 7a Comparison of the excretory systems of Carcinus *and* Astacus.

Figure 7b Concentration of the urine in different parts of the excretory system of Astacus.

10.5.1 Osmoregulation in insects

The insects present a very interesting but rather unusual picture. Their anatomy and physiology are essentially water conservative and in this they are well adapted for a terrestrial existence. The cuticle has a waxy layer which is impermeable to water; the respiratory surfaces are internal and may be guarded by valves (Unit 6; Section 6.3); the excretory product is uric acid. Insects lay shelled eggs. Thus, in design terms, they are geared to resist desiccation.

The excretory product being primarily uric acid, the excretory demand on water may not be great; the system by which it is excreted is quite unlike anything we have discussed so far. A large number of blind-ending ducts arise from the gut at the point where the mid-gut becomes the hind-gut; these ducts are called Malpighian tubules, and they are bathed in the blood which circulates in the body cavity (Unit 5). The tubules secrete a urine, which flows into the hind-gut. Before the urine emerges with the faeces, it passes the rectal glands, which withdraw water from the urine/faeces mixture. These glands also remove a large percentage of the salts (mainly potassium) from the urine.

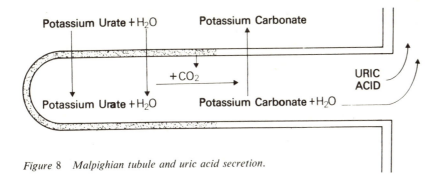

Figure 8 *Malpighian tubule and uric acid secretion.*

Would it be fair to say that there is an analogy between this system and the vertebrate nephron, with the Malpighian tubules corresponding to the glomerulus and the rectal gland to the distal tubule and collecting ducts?

The analogy is not really a good one because there is no ultrafiltration into the Malpighian tubules, the urine is actively secreted into the lumen by the cells of the tube. This means that the urine does not have the same constitution as the plasma of the blood because selection has entered into the process of secretion. In the vertebrate kidney the glomerular filtrate is virtually identical with the blood except that it is almost protein free (only molecules with a molecular weight of less than 67 000 cross the filter).

It was first suggested by Wigglesworth in 1931 that the blood-sucking bug *Rhodnius* produced uric acid by actively secreting soluble urates, probably potassium urate, into the distal (blind) end of the tubule. (You will recall seeing both Sir Vincent Wigglesworth and *Rhodnius* in the TV programme of Unit 9.) Further along the tubule, nearer the gut, the secretion of CO_2 occurs, which acidifies the contents, causing the precipitation of uric acid crystals which are then carried into the gut (Fig. 8). Water and potassium are reabsorbed from the faeces/urine mixture by the rectal glands.

uric acid secretion

Subsequent work has suggested that something like this scheme applies to most insect Malphigian tubules, though the ion involved is not always potassium. It is most interesting to see how this system is adapted to life in different environments.

(a) Terrestrial environments, with ample water

herbivorous insects

The stick insect, *Carausius* is a herbivore which feeds continuously on fresh plant material. Thus it has a good supply of dietary water available to it, and a large surplus of potassium (plants have a high potassium level compared with that of most animal tissues). Urine production by the Malphigian tubules is rapid— the equivalent of all the body water is secreted every 24 hours and the equivalent of all the potassium every 3 hours. Thus the tubules are doing a rather similar job, in this respect, to the mammalian glomeruli. The urine is hypo-osmotic to the blood (see Table 2), and extensive water and salt reabsorption takes place through the rectal gland, the final fluid being more than twice as concentrated as the blood.

Notice, in Table 2, the very high degree of osmotic concentration (and therefore, presumably, osmotic work) achieved by the rectal glands, producing a fluid with double the osmotic pressure of the plasma. Although this does not compare impressively with the performance of the desert rat quoted in Moffat (p. 5) (blood 300 mOsm; urine 6 000 mOsm), it is not necessary that it should.

17

Table 2 Concentrations (mM/l) of some of the contents of the plasma, urine and rectal fluid of the stick insect

Substance	Plasma	Urine emerging from tubules	Rectal fluid after action by glands
Sodium	11	5	19
Potassium	18	145	320
Chloride	87	65	—
Uric acid	0.27	2.6	—
Total osmotic pressure in mOsm/l	320	317	735

Why not?

Because the insect excretes uric acid, which precipitates in strong concentrations and does not exert a very high osmotic pressure. Also, because water is not in very short supply.

Thus the animal is an efficient water conserver and, given the relatively constant availability of water and proportional intake of salts provided by the diet, it is well adapted. However, it does not cope well with an experimental loading of the tissues with either salts or water; the rectal glands normally reabsorb 80 per cent of the potassium produced by the tubules and the majority of the water, and they are unable to vary this quickly. Thus, if the animal is experimentally loaded with salt or water, it may take several days to excrete the excess; but, as the animal is basically waterproof and obviously not given to going on unnecessary drinking bouts, such loading will not normally occur.

moist food

(b) *Terrestrial environment with little water*

The mealworm *Tenebrio molitor* is an animal which may live in an environment with little or no free water; this is especially true of the larvae, which live on flour. The mealworm larva has an acute problem of water conservation. The blood osmotic concentration is high (520 mOsm in the adult), and the animal even has the ability to take up some water from humid air. The removal of water from the faeces and urine by the rectal gland is truly remarkable—indeed, it is almost total, leaving a dry pellet of faeces and uric acid with a notional osmotic pressure of 13 000 mOsm, twice that of the urine of the desert rat!

dry food

(c) *Terrestrial environment with the water intake very variable*

There *are* some insects that do go on drinking bouts; for example, blood-sucking parasites such as *Rhodnius*. During long periods of fast, *Rhodnius* must resist desiccation, as many other insects do, but when it feeds it takes on a relatively enormous amount of fluid—so much that it becomes virtually immobile. Thus, equally, it must have some means of varying the common pattern we mentioned above. You saw what it does in the TV programme of Unit 9; although how the hormone acts to produce the increase in tubular urine flow is not yet fully worked out.

The tubular function differs slightly from that shown in Figure 8, in that although most of the urate secretion occurs at the distal end, as shown, there is considerable reabsorption of water in the proximal region of the tubule. It is possible that this part of the mechanism is affected by the diuretic hormone that Dr Maddrell described in the TV programme of Unit 9. The rectal glands are quite small but, supported by tubular reabsorption, they are adequate for water conservation during the slow part of the digestion of a blood meal or while fasting. During the periods of sudden water intake, as you saw, the stretching of the stomach triggers neuro-secretion and the release of a diuretic hormone from the mesothoracic ganglion, with the result that very large quantities of urine are released.

blood feeders

(d) Freshwater environment

The larva of the mosquito *Aedes aegypti*, the yellow-fever mosquito, lives in freshwater. (You may recall seeing mosquito larvae in the TV programme of Unit 6.) Thus it will tend to gain water by osmosis and, if it produces urine to counteract this, it will lose salts by excretion in addition to any loss by diffusion. However, it has a cuticle with a low permeability and breathes air, so the problem is not as great as that faced by freshwater fish. However, the rectal gland re-absorbs salts from the urine to produce an excretory flow which is hypo-osmotic to the blood, and the anal papillae absorb salt from the water against the osmotic gradient.

aquatic insects

(e) Marine environment

The mosquito *Aedes detritus* has a larva that lives in sea or brackish water, though it is able to tolerate freshwater and even water more concentrated than sea water (Fig. 6). In freshwater (Table 3), it behaves much as *Aedes aegypti*, although the anal papillae are almost vestigial. In sea water, the blood concentration rises (Table 3) and the rectal glands reabsorb water as in the terrestrial forms—you will notice the concentration of the rectal fluid lies between that of the stick insect and the mealworm.

marine environment

Table 3 Concentration of the blood and rectal fluid (in mOsm/l) of *Aedes detritus* in fresh and sea water

Medium	Blood	Rectal fluid
Freshwater	194	112
Sea water (940 mOsm/l)	322	1 060

There is some evidence that the animal behaves rather like a marine teleost, in that it may drink sea water to make up the water lost by osmosis. Whether the surplus salt is excreted in the concentrated rectal fluid or by special sodium secretory cells elsewhere is not known.

These examples illustrate something of the way insects adapt to differing osmotic situations, and also some of the similarities and differences between the ways these problems are solved by insects and by other groups. These examples also raise a point that previous ones did not. If you return to Table 2 (p. 17), you will see that it reveals a very thought-provoking group of facts. The urine is *hypo-osmotic* to the plasma, although the ionic concentration is higher. How can it happen that proportionately *more* water gets into the tubules than is in the plasma? A similar question arises again with the rectal fluid, in this case in reverse. How is water apparently preferentially removed *against* a large osmotic gradient? Some parts of the Malphigian tubules (the proximal parts) have been shown to be capable of producing urine no less than 40 mOsm hypo-osmotic to the plasma. So far, these data and others relating to the electrical charges on either side of the membranes have been satisfactorily explained only on the basis of the active transport of water. This is very interesting, because many physiologists deny that this phenomenon is possible, and it is certainly not thought to occur in vertebrates.

10.5.2 Unicellular animals

An obvious place to study osmoregulation at a cellular level would seem to be in protozoans, but fundamental answers have not yet emerged from such studies.

Marine unicellular animals are isosmotic with their environment; those living in freshwater clearly are not. Many freshwater species have a visible water pump, the *contractile vacuole*. (You saw it in action in the TV programme of S100 Unit 18.) This vacuole fills quite rapidly with fluid when the animal is in fresh-

contractile vacuole

19

water, and then bursts, releasing the water to the outside. The vacuole is not excretory, its function is osmoregulation. At first sight this seems to be a satisfactory answer to the question: how does a single cell osmoregulate? However, it merely moves the fundamental problem one step in from the cell membrane. To be of value to the animal in maintaining its osmolality, the fluid in the vacuole, would need to be hypo-osmotic. If it were isosmotic, the process might prevent the cell bursting, but would rapidly leach it of all its salts. This would mean that Na pumps in the cell membrane would have to pick up salt from the freshwater (where they may be very dilute indeed) as fast as the vacuole pumped them out—a very dubious hypothesis.

If, on the other hand, the fluid in the vacuole *is* hypo-osmotic, how can this be? The active transport of water without ion movement is an idea much frowned on by most physiologists, though it has been demonstrated in insects. If the water follows Na pumped into the vacuole by Na pumps, what then happens to the Na? Can it be withdrawn again leaving the water behind? Is the vacuole membrane waterproof? Electron micrographs show many mitochondria around the vacuole and a rather unusual, dense, membrane—but the questions remain unanswered. It is quite likely that when we know how contractile vacuoles really work we may know something of osmoregulation by the membranes of cells without contractile vacuoles—e.g. *Hydra*.

Summary

The first part of the Unit considered the types of environment—marine, freshwater and terrestrial—and the relationship between these environments and various groups of animals. The fact was stressed that marine invertebrates may need to regulate the relative concentration of particular ions, even though osmoregulation is unnecessary. The problems of migration from the sea to a dilute medium were then stressed, and the theoretically possible solutions discussed. The next Section (10.2), a very brief Section, discussed the relationship between the excretory product and the availability of water. The mammalian kidney was described in the set text, which should have been read at this point. Questions on the operation of the kidney were asked; you should have been able to answer these from the text and your memory of Unit 6.

An extremely brief account of the secretion and action of ADH, aldosterone and renin then followed. After this we left the mammalian mechanism and considered the solutions adopted by freshwater teleosts, marine teleosts and elasmobranchs.

Finally, some invertebrate solutions to these problems were considered. The ways in which different crustaceans respond to changes in the environment were mentioned, and some of the mechanisms employed by insects to osmoregulate in different environments were described. The Unit ended on the unsolved problem of the contractile vacuole.

Self-assessment Questions

SAQ 1 (*Objectives 1 and 3, Sections 10.3 and 10.4*) What is meant by ultra-filtration? Is it essential to survival in teleost fish?

SAQ 2 (*Objectives 3 and 6, Section 10.3*) What factors determine the minimum urine flow in a mammal deprived of water?

SAQ 3 (*Objectives 5 and 6, Section 10.3.2*) A man may drink 7 litres of beer in 3 hours in a pub. At the end of this time will his blood be significantly more dilute than at the beginning?

SAQ 4 (*Objectives 5 and 6, Section 10.3*) If you placed clamps which reduced the blood flow by 75 per cent on the renal arteries of a mammal for 2 hours, what effects might you expect to see after their removal on (a) the rate of filtration, and (b) rate of sodium excretion.

SAQ 5 (*Objectives 2 and 3, Sections 10.1, 10.4, 10.5*) Compare the processes of osmoregulation in the freshwater crustacean *Astacus* with those of a trout in freshwater. Do you consider that they differ in principle?

Self-assessment Answers and Comments

SAQ 1 Ultra filtration is the process whereby a liquid is forced across a filtering membrane by a pressure difference. It is essential to the survival of most freshwater teleosts, in order that the kidney may remove sufficient water from the blood. It is not essential for marine teleosts, or migratory teleosts in sea water. Some teleosts thought to be aglomerular inhabit freshwater—it is not known how they survive.

SAQ 2 Such a mammal will be secreting the maximum amount of ADH, but the urine flow cannot be reduced to zero because there will be urea in the glomerular filtrate, which will exert an osmotic pull and therefore require water to be excreted with it. The amount of urea will be one of the determining factors. Another factor will be the state of 'salt-loading'. If there is surplus Na in the body, aldosterone release will be inhibited and salt (and thus water) will be excreted. Another factor is the anatomy of the kidney of the particular animal concerned.

SAQ 3 Yes it will. 7 litres an hour (a real figure by the way) is about 40 cm³/minute. The maximum diuresis (i.e. *no* ADH) is 20 cm³/min, unless the GFR is increased (and dilute alcohol does not have much effect on GFR), and the beer will be absorbed quite fast from the gut. Thus, there will be some 'water intoxication' caused by the dilution of the plasma, in addition to any effects of the alcohol on the central nervous system.

SAQ 4 The reduction in blood pressure to the kidneys will stimulate the release of renin. This will act via angiotensin I and II to raise blood pressure and stimulate aldosterone secretion.

Therefore (a) GFR will increase temporarily (b) sodium excretion (or, at least, concentration) will be reduced.

SAQ 5 Both animals have a relatively impermeable integument; both take up water by osmosis through the respiratory surfaces; both remove fluid from the body in a urine produced by ultra-filtration; both have a lower plasma osmolality than their marine relatives. Thus, although their anatomy is entirely different, the solutions they have adopted to the situation they share are very similar.

Acknowledgements

Grateful acknowledgement is made to the following sources for material used in this unit:

Fig. 4 Cambridge University Press for E. Baldwin, *Introduction to Comparative Physiology*, 1949; *Fig. 5* Physiological Reviews for E. Marshall, *Physiological Reviews*, Vol. 14, 1934; *Figs. 6 and 7a* Cambridge University Press for J. A. Ramsay, *Physiological approach to the lower animals* 1952; *Fig. 7b* Springer-Verlag for H. Peters, *Z. Morph. Okol. Tiere*. Vol. 30, 1935; *Fig. 8* Cambridge University Press for V. B. Wigglesworth, *J. Exp. Biol*. Vol. 8, 1931; Table 2 Cambridge University Press for V. B. Wigglesworth, *J. Exp. Biol*. Vol. 32, 1955 and Vol. 33, 1956.

Physiological Mechanisms and
Physiological Evolution
Unit 11

Contents

Table A

List of Scientific Terms, Concepts and Principles used in Unit 11

Taken as prerequisites			Introduced in this Unit			
1 **Assumed from** **general knowledge**	**2** **Introduced in** **previous Unit**	**Unit** **No.**	**3** **Developed in this Unit or** **in its set book(s)**	**Page** **No.**	**4** **Developed in a** **later Unit**	**Unit** **No.**
	All items listed in Table A of Units 1 to 10		growth patterns of vertebrates	9		
			annual and seasonal cycles	13		
			hibernation	14		
			diapause	15		
			poisonous substances in plants and insects	17		
			factors controlling the reproductive cycle of the rabbit flea	18		
			interactions between internal parasites and hosts	21		

Objectives

After you have studied this Unit you should be able to:

1 Define or recognize the meaning of terms in Table A.

2 List at least five major differences in structural organization between terrestrial plants, represented by angiosperms, and terrestrial animals, represented by mammals and insects, and to relate these differences to physiological differences which ultimately are derived from differences in type of nutrition.

(SAQ 1.)

3 Give 3 examples of convergent physiological evolution among unrelated* organisms.

4 Give 3 examples of similar physiological responses by unrelated organisms to variation in external environmental factors.

5 Give 3 examples of the evolution of interrelated physiological mechanisms by unrelated organisms.

(ITQs and SAQs 2 and 3.)

6 Apply the principles given in this Unit to relevant situations or information not dealt with in the Unit text.

(ITQs and SAQ 3.)

---

* Unrelated is taken here to mean organisms separated taxonomically at least at the level of Class.

This final Unit is intended to act as revision for earlier Units by making generalizations that set information already available to you within new frames of reference. You are therefore advised to read the whole Unit if you can.

Differences at the cellular level are considered first, in Section 11.1; the principal contrast is in nutrition with and without green plastids. Then, in Section 11.2, we proceed to differences at the whole organism level, contrasting plants and animals that live on land and relating many of the remarkable differences between them to the fundamental difference in nutrition. These two Sections are straightforward, depending on earlier Units and general knowledge.

Sections 11.3 and 11.4 deal with adaptation between organisms and their environments. The influence of physical and chemical factors is studied in Section 11.3, mainly through relationships between growth and reproduction of plants and animals and climatic changes in the British Isles. Similar cues are used by unrelated groups of organisms that show similar annual cycles. You could omit part of this Section (see the Study Comment) if short of time. Interactions with other species that live in the same environment often involve physiological adjustments between unrelated organisms; three examples are studied in Section 11.4. You could omit Sections 11.4.1 and 11.4.3 which both include new information, but you are advised at least to skim through 11.4.2 because this account of rabbit flea physiology is intended as revision of parts of Units 8 and 9.

The final Section discusses the evolution of physiological mechanisms by considering whether hypotheses about the evolution of animals, discussed in Unit 1, are supported by the information given in subsequent Units. The Section refers to Appendix I, which consists of summaries of some aspects of Units 4, 5, 6, 8, 9 and 10; you are advised at least to read these.

There is no prescribed reading for this Unit and no Home Experiment.

11.0 Introduction

> When we no longer look at an organic being as a savage looks at a ship, as something wholly beyond his comprehension; when we regard every production of nature as one which has had a long history; when we contemplate every complex structure and instinct as the summing up of many contrivances, each useful to its possessor, in the same way as any great mechanical invention is the summing up of the labour, the experience, the reason, and even the blunders of numerous workmen; when we thus view each organic being, how far more interesting,—I speak from experience,—does the study of natural history become. (Charles Darwin, *Origin of Species.*)

This Course has concentrated to a large extent on how living organisms 'work' and on making comparisons between different kinds of living organisms. As a background to this study, the first two Units included surveys of the Animal and Plant Kingdoms; these were concerned with the characteristic structure of members of the higher order taxa and also indicated how these taxa might be arranged in scales of complexity. For plants, types of life history and adaptations to terrestrial life (as contrasted with aquatic life) were discussed in some detail. For animals, a tentative phylogenetic 'shrub' was constructed, based on types of body cavity and of movement.

Now that you have come to the last Unit, it seems appropriate to consider the physiology that you have studied against the background of structural adaptation and phylogeny and to try to fit the detailed material that you have met into a coherent whole. In doing this, we shall refer to material in earlier Units so we shall be helping you to revise them as well as to organize the information within different frames of reference.

The Course has dealt with multicellular organisms almost exclusively so it is logical first, in Section 11.1, to consider whether we can make any generalizations based on comparing their component cells. From this, in Section 11.2, we proceed to study whole organisms, dealing mainly with the contrasts between terrestrial plants and terrestrial animals. In the next Section (11.3), observations on how physiological changes in plants and animals are related to changes in environment are brought together by considering how the annual climatic changes in the British Isles affect the lives of organisms. The following Section (11.4) deals with some interactions between organisms of different taxa living in the same community, showing how physiological processes in one species of organism may have evolved in special and highly specific relation to physiological features of an unrelated species.

The Course concludes (Section 11.5) with a discussion of whether physiological mechanisms provide a good basis for constructing probable lines of evolution for the Animal Kingdom.

11.1 Eucaryotic Cells with and without Plastids

Study comment

This short Section deals with physiological mechanisms at the level of cells that are components of multicellular organisms.

All living organisms are cellular; that is, the bodies of simple and complex living organisms are built up of discrete units of living material. Each (eucaryotic) unit is bounded by a membrane surrounding cytoplasm and a nucleus (see S100* , Unit 14, for a discussion of the cell theory and Units 1 and 2 of this Course). The procaryotic cell is in a different category, and it is excluded from all that follows. Two broad patterns of cellular organization and anatomy commonly occur, cells with plastids and cells without, corresponding to two Kingdoms—Plants and Animals.

Apart from the basic question of nutrition, both types of cell appear to have much in common as far as their physiological 'mechanisms' are concerned and this is

* *The Open University (1971) S100* Science: A Foundation Course, *The Open University Press.*

7

reflected in or is a consequence of the similarity of their subcellular and molecular structure. For instance, low molecular weight material enters both types of cells by diffusion and by an active transport system. Materials leave both types of cells by similar physiological mechanisms. Movement within cells happens as a result of microcirculation in the cytoplasm (see Units 3, 5 and 6) and as a result of diffusion.

Tissue respiration occurs in similar organelles in plant and animal cells, involving enzymes whose chemistry and physical properties are similar. Leaving aside photosynthesis as a very special case, cellular synthesis, like cellular respiration, cannot be sensibly categorized as either plant-like or animal-like because, as far as is known, the biochemical processes are similar—although there are important differences in the end products—notably the synthesis of lignin by plant cells (see Unit 2).   **respiration**

cellular synthesis

Against this wide range of similarities there is one outstanding difference between the two Kingdoms which can be referred to the cellular organization—nutrition.   **nutrition**
Some cells in plants contain green plastids. These cells may be able to photosynthesize. Some plant cells and most animal cells lack green plastids and so are unable to photosynthesize (S100, Units 15–16, and Unit 3 in this Course). The effect of this in terms of whole organisms was discussed in S100, Unit 20, and Units 1 and 3 of this Course (autotrophes and heterotrophes).

11.2   Plants and Animals

Study comment

Starting from the nutritional differences that arise from the presence or absence of plastids in their cells, the very considerable differences in structure and habit between terrestrial plants (represented by angiosperms) and animals (represented by mammals and insects) are surveyed. The information in this Section is either derived from earlier Units or should be general knowledge. Read through it fairly fast if you are short of time.

11.2.1   Mobility and skeletons

A successful land-living organism must be able to obtain all its requirements from its surroundings and it must be able to withstand the physical and chemical changes in its surroundings. Given the ability to photosynthesize, then the prime requirements are light, supplies of carbon dioxide, oxygen, water and mineral salts, and space. Because light and the atmospheric gases are equally available over the whole of the land surface, there would seem to be no particular selective advantage in mobility (see Fig. 1). If, however, as is the case with the animals, metabolizable molecules must be captured rather than synthesized, then mobility could be advantageous—unless, of course, such molecules were equally available all over the land surface, which is not the case.

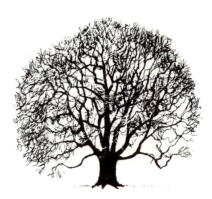

Figure 1   *An oak* Quercus *in winter as an example of a large terrestrial plant.*

If mobility is advantageous, it seems to follow that sense organs, in particular distance receptors such as eyes and ears, a brain and a nervous system are necessary (see Fig. 2). Similarly mobility on land seems almost always associated with possession of muscles, some sort of skeleton and a rapid internal transport system. On the other hand, the photosynthetic plant, immobile in its surroundings, can 'dispense' with these while being subject to selection pressures favouring completely different anatomical solutions. The development of a root and shoot system leading to the efficient acquisition of water and salts from the soil is inconceivable in mobile organisms. The development of a non-jointed skeleton rather than a jointed skeleton system is obviously more efficient for non-mobile organisms. The green plants' ability to synthesize lignin is crucial. But given this, the subsequent development of hollow supporting cells in a ring—so typical of all shoot systems—can be seen again as efficient utilization of supporting material, since hollow cylinders can support greater loads imposing bending stress as well as compression than similar weights of the same material built into solid cylinders. Notice the parallelism here between hollow stelar systems, exoskeletons and some bones of vertebrates.

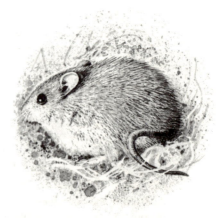

Figure 2   *A fieldmouse* Apodemus *as an example of a mammal that lives in oakwoods.*

11.2.2 Circulation

Transport within a body supported by hollow fluid-filled cylinders permeable to water is almost certain provided that evaporation can take place from the upper end of the system: in the case of green plants this is inevitable anyway since thin permeable surfaces are essential to allow for the gaseous exchanges upon which photosynthesis depends (see Unit 3). Hence, although multicellular animals and plants both incorporate circulatory systems, those in animals almost always depend on muscular contractions of part of the system, whereas in plants upward transport in the transpiration stream does not involve muscles or the expenditure of metabolic energy. It is necessary here to distinguish between upward transpirational movement of water plus dissolved salts and the maintenance of the system by which continuous entry of water into the root is effected even when there is no transpiration. Water uptake (see Unit 2) is almost certainly a process that requires metabolic energy.

Translocation of sugars and amino acids through the plant body is achieved principally in the phloem system (see Unit 3) and is based on a different prime mover from either transpiration or muscle cells. It may be that phloem transport will eventually be shown to depend upon changes in space of protein macromolecules. If so, then interesting similarities between translocation and some animal prime movers may be seen.

11.2.3 Shape, size and life span

Stemming from the radical differences in support system, there are differences in overall growth size and life span of plants and animals. Plants grow as the result of either apical, intercalary or lateral meristems (Unit 7). In animals in general, growth is not the prerogative of localized parts of the body, although some structures may have localized areas of growth such as the epiphyses of mammalian bones. If growth did occur in localized parts mobility might well be severely and adversely affected. Arthropods can only grow in volume when the exoskeleton is shed; their mobility is reduced and the animals are nearly helpless until the new exoskeleton has hardened. They grow in weight between moults as well as during a moult.

Because the lignified mature cells of the support system are dead, growth in height in plants can occur only in non-lignified areas, e.g. at the apices of stem and root (Unit 7). Provided the meristematic cells retain their capacity to divide and do not differentiate, the shape, size and length of life of the individual may be indefinite. In each of these three features animals are sharply distinct from green plants. Generally terrestrial animals grow to a characteristic adult size and shape and stop growing. The lives of terrestrial animals are generally short, from a few weeks to a few years, but some plants may live for more than a thousand years while others live for a few weeks only.

The general situation amongst mammals and birds is that juveniles grow rather quickly until they reach the size of their parents. While at or near this size the juvenile matures to become the reproductively mature adult; then for the rest of its life it maintains its size within narrow limits (see Fig. 3).

Whales and fish show a quite different pattern. In these two groups, although the shape of the juvenile stages is very similar to that of adult stages (see Fig. 4), size is much more variable even when maturity is reached. 'The older the animal, the bigger it is' appears to be the general rule in these two groups—in this respect, whales and fish are almost plant-like!

Having made these general statements, it must be admitted straight away that there are some obvious constraints which operate. For instance, size and shape are often determined in part genetically. Consequently dwarf individuals and giant individuals occur (in plants and in animals) as well as individuals of abnormal shape. In addition there are mechanical constraints. Above or below a particular size, movement, for instance, may be impeded or impossible. This aspect was discussed in connection with birds and bird flight in S100, Unit 21. The dynamics of swimming and the demands the physical properties of the environment make on aquatic animals may explain the constancy of shape but not variability in size in the whales and fish.

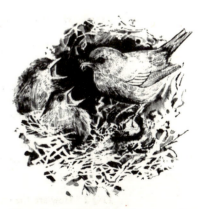

Figure 3 Adult robin feeding young that have just left the nest.

muscular circulatory systems

transpiration

phloem

growth patterns

9

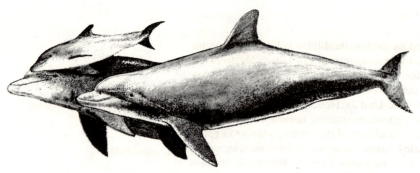

Figure 4   Bottle-nosed dolphin about 3·5 m long with newly born young.

In the water, size limits may be governed not so much by mechanical considerations but by the availability of food and/or by the increasing chances of crippling or fatal happenings associated with a long life. For instance, the accumulation of parasites may, even if the yearly rate of infection is low, at the end of a long life ensure that a host carries so big a burden of parasites that its efficiency drops with fatal consequences. In this connection, it is interesting to note that in woody plants the bulk of their bodies are dead anyway—and perhaps accidental injury is less likely to be fatal—but the dead tissue is probably preserved by accumulation of substances with antibiotic properties, such as tannins (see later). In animals, the bulk of their tissue is made of living cells even in senile individuals; damage to living tissues anywhere in the animal body may have severe repercussions affecting the efficiency of the whole organism.

parasites

living and dead cells

11.2.4   Sex and reproduction

For both plants and animals, sexual reproduction on land presents problems when compared with sexual reproduction in the sea. Many animal and plant cells are isosmotic with seawater so gametes released into the sea can survive for quite long periods of time, and male gametes can find those of opposite sex by swimming, usually by ciliary activity. Seaweeds, many marine invertebrates and teleost fishes release gametes into the sea. Delicate unprotected gametes cannot survive in air (or for more than a fraction of a minute in fresh waters because of osmotic problems) so discharge of unprotected gametes on land could not be effective.

gametes

As pointed out in Unit 2, the development of an enclosed and protected female gametophyte can be seen as a necessary part of land colonization by plants.

ITQ 1   How are the gametes brought together in angiosperms?

Read the answer to ITQ 1 (p. 29).

Angiosperm sporophytes are rooted plants; sexual reproduction with cross-fertilization is made possible by the production of resistant spores that can each grow into a male gametophyte when very close to the protected female gametophyte, the ovule inside the ovary. There are adaptive differences in structure between the flowers of insect-pollinated and wind-pollinated plants; these must have arisen by variation acted upon by natural selection.

pollination

ITQ 2   How are the gametes brought together in mammals and insects?

Read the answer to ITQ 2 (p. 29).

Copulation between a pair of mobile animals is only possible if there is mutual recognition and at least a minimum of co-operative behaviour. Both mammals and insects have courtship and mating rituals, sometimes quite elaborate; among vertebrates, the most spectacular courtship displays are those of some birds. Freshwater teleosts often also have elaborate mating behaviour; some of these fish are viviparous, with internal fertilization.

courtship

10

There are clearly many contrasts between the reproductive mechanisms of terrestrial plants and animals. Typically the animals are either male or female but the sporophyte generation of angiosperms is usually capable of producing both male and female spores in flowers that typically have both stamens and ovaries. Asexual reproduction and forms of crypto-sexual reproduction (e.g. apomixis*) are common in plants. Some insects reproduce by parthenogenesis§ but most insects and all vertebrates reproduce only by a sexual process. Some plants have elaborate floral mechanisms that prevent self-fertilization and allow only a few species of animals to act as pollinators, carrying male spores to female parts of flowers. Mobile animals have no need to rely on go-betweens for transmission of gametes, but internal parasites often have one or more intermediate hosts through which larval stages are dispersed and reach new hosts. Some animals actively seek members of their own species and live in groups but 'pure stands' of plants are the result either of some form of asexual reproduction or of many seeds reaching the same locality by chance and growing there successfully.

asexual and sexual reproduction

11.2.5 Sensory systems and co-ordination

The absence of recognizable sense organs in green plants and their basic importance in the lives of animals already referred to does not mean that plants lack sensitivity to their surroundings or their internal environments. The integration of growth in general and flowering in particular (discussed in Unit 7) and the regulation of stomatal aperture (discussed in Unit 3) are examples of reactivity which imply the presence and operation of sensitive cells or tissues. Integration of response is achieved via hormones in both animals and plants, plus nervous systems in animals. It would seem plausible that the absence of nerves is attributable to an absence of a positive selective advantage to plants of a relatively high-speed co-ordination system. Similarly the absence of a memory store and brain system, the absence both of learning and the ability to modify reactions to stimuli (a set of widespread properties among animals) can be correlated with the lack of mobility in plants plus the plastic responses of plants. For whereas animals can avoid and/or evade adverse environmental situations, plants appear to be able to tolerate adverse situations or respond, usually by growth, in a limited but suitable manner.

nerves and hormones

11.2.6 Regulation

Regulation of behaviour is only one aspect of regulation. Animals in general regulate many (or several) parameters of their internal environment. For instance, regulation of pH of body fluids (Unit 9), regulation of water content (Unit 10), and regulation by excretion of metabolic waste products (Unit 10). The organ systems involved, although varying in detail of anatomy and physiological mode of operation are generally classed together as 'kidneys'. By contrast, green plants lack organized kidney-type systems.

Animals need to dispose of massive amounts of nitrogenous excretory material; this follows from their dependence on exogenous protein sources. Usually the amino-acid composition of the diet is different from that of the body and an excess of some must be consumed and absorbed to allow ingestion of sufficient quantities of other essential amino acids. The excess of ingested nitrogen over that needed by the body plus any nitrogenous breakdown products of metabolism are generally got rid of by excretion; in some animals, small quantities may be transformed into substances that are stored, such as some of the nitrogenous pigments of butterflies' wings.

nitrogenous excretion

Plants synthesize their own proteins from amino acids that they synthesize from inorganic compounds and sugars. It is probable that cellular reactions can be regulated so that little protein is produced in excess of that needed for growth and replacement of cells. Thus plants should have no problem of disposal of

---

* Apomixis occurs when seeds are produced without any fertilization process. In roses and currants, seed is formed by cells outside the embryo sac which are part of the sporophyte generation; in some plants, the process is a type of parthenogenesis with the seed formed by spore mother cells or unfertilized gametes.

§ See Glossary of Zoological Terms in the Invertebrate Survey.

excess of nitrogenous compounds. However, plants do produce 'waste' materials: probably most of these are synthesized into complex substances that may make the plant distasteful or poisonous to animals (see Section 11.4.1). Deciduous trees in autumn withdraw much of the protein from their leaves, which senesce and fall; nevertheless, these fallen leaves provide quite a rich source of nitrogen for specialized organisms (in the 'litter') that consume them and break them down (refer back to S100, Unit 20).

plant 'waste' substances

Regulation of water content by means of a kidney or kidney analogue appears to be an activity characteristic of animals. Green plants lack separate systems with a water-regulating function but many have structural adaptations that reduce water loss. It seems likely that evaporative loss of water from the stems and leaves and absorption via the roots balance over a range of water contents tolerated by the plants' tissues.

11.2.7 Conclusions

It is perhaps as well at this stage to be clear that questions of comparative efficiency—e.g. are animals more efficient than plants?—are meaningless in such a general form. If the question is made more specific—are land plants more efficient than land animals? for example—it is made no more meaningful simply because there is no possibility of forming an answer. But it should be clear that there are considerable similarities at the metabolic, subcellular and cellular levels. Yet it is the small differences at these lower levels that account for most of the striking differences that we can observe at the organism level. Whether one chooses to pay more attention to the similarities or more attention to the differences depends on the context of the discussion.

11.3 Physiological Mechanisms and Environment

Study comment

Physiological adaptation to different environments is treated briefly by reference to earlier Units; the bulk of the Section concerns the mechanisms by which physiological cycles in plants and animals are related to climatic changes. Much of this is revision of material in Units 7 and 8; 'diapause' (in insects) is a mechanism new to you that you could omit if short of time.

Organisms do not exist in isolation from the rest of the world. They live in definite environments where they are subject to physical and chemical factors and interact with the other organisms present (refer to S100, Unit 20). It is not surprising that physiological evolution has been influenced by physical, chemical and biotic factors of the environment. The conditions in many different environments are discussed in Course S2-3*, Environment, but there are some aspects of physiological adaptation that have been studied in this Course.

Recall some examples of physiological adaptations that have been evolved in more than one group of organisms by answering the following questions:

> **ITQ 3** What problems of life on land (as contrasted with life in water) affect both plants and animals?
>
> **ITQ 4** What osmotic problems are faced by all animals that live in fresh waters? Give at least one example of similar solutions to these problems evolved by animals of different phyla.
>
> **ITQ 5** What excretory problems are faced by terrestrial animals that live under dry conditions? What nitrogenous excretory product is produced by both birds and insects?
>
> *Read the answers to ITQ 3, 4 and 5.*

life on land and in water

Some environments scarcely vary through the year and even remain the same by day and night; examples are the depths of the oceans and deep caves. But it is characteristic of most environments that there is variation, usually of a fairly regular pattern. Generally there is a contrast between day and night. You heard

* *The Open University (1972) S2-3 Environment: A Second Level Course, The Open University Press.*

in Radio programme 2 about *circadian rhythms*, illustrated by observations on cockroaches and on man. Similar rhythms have been observed in many groups of animals, such as fish and crabs, active either by day or by night, and also in some plants, such as daisies whose flowers close at night and open the next morning. The stimuli that trigger off these rhythms are generally light and/or darkness but temperature changes may also play a part. Some rhythms are 'endogenous' but others are controlled entirely by the external changes so the organism is arhythmic in a uniform environment.

> Suggest other types of regular change in environment that might be associated with periodicity of physiological function in organisms.

You probably thought of the *annual* changes in temperature and light that occur in temperate and polar zones. These were mentioned in S100, Unit 20. Here are other examples:

1 *Tidal* changes affect organisms living on seashores and in shallow seas. On most coasts there are two high tides and two low tides every day, but a single tidal cycle is just under 12 hours so the times of high and low tide alter in a regular way. The organisms on the shore are exposed to quite different conditions when covered by the sea or when the tide is out; most of them are active when the tide is in and inactive when the tide goes out.

2 *Lunar* changes occur because the moon waxes and wanes over a period of approximately 28 days. The phases of the moon affect the height of tides and so add an extra type of periodic change to tidal cycles, with 'spring' tides occurring just after full and new moon and 'neap' tides after the first and third quarters. The contrast at night between periods of full and new moon is very obvious to those living in country districts.

3 Changes in *rainfall*, leading to regular dry and wet seasons, are common in many parts of the world, including tropical areas; examples are the 'monsoons' affecting India and much of SE Asia. These climatic patterns result from regular changes in patterns of atmospheric pressure.

You can read about adaptations to life on the sea-shore and to tidal changes in Course S2–3, Environment, Block 2. Lunar rhythms have been postulated for many organisms, including women; there is no connection, however, between menstruation and phases of the moon. Many marine organisms have regular spawning cycles related to the moon but investigation of these involves distinguishing between the effects of spring tides and those of the full moon. The sea-urchin *Centrechinus setosus* (Fig. 5), from the Red Sea, continued to display a cycle of gonad growth and to spawn at the full moon even when held in wooden boxes (in the dark) floating at the surface of the sea (to exclude the tidal effect). This urchin appears to have an endogenous 28-day rhythm. Synchronization of spawning cycles is likely to be of great survival value to sessile or sedentary animals that shed eggs and sperm into the sea, relying on 'chance' encounters between them for continuation of the species. One of the more famous instances of remarkable synchronization is the breeding of the Palolo worm (Fig. 6), a polychaete that lives in Pacific coral reefs. These worms shed the posterior part of the body, full of eggs or sperm, at the last quarter of the moon in October and November every year. These shed parts wriggle towards the surface as the sun rises and the natives of some of these Islands traditionally collect as much as they can and hold a 'Feast of the Rising Worm'. So far the physiological bases for these examples of lunar periodicity have not been elucidated.

Annual and seasonal cycles associated with the dramatic changes in light and temperature of high latitudes and with regular alternations of dry and wet seasons have been investigated for many animals and plants.

> Recall examples quoted in this Course (in Units 7 and 8).

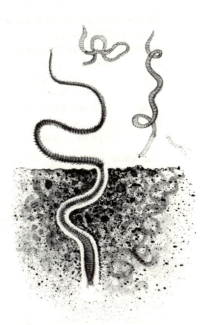

Figure 5 *The sea-urchin* Centrechinus setosus.

Figure 6 *The Palolo worm* Leodice fucata: *mature worm shedding the posterior end of its body and shed parts swimming in the sea.*

Flowering in certain plants, e.g. chrysanthemums, spinach, winter wheat; reproductive cycles in many mammals, e.g. sheep, deer.

In both these sets of examples, environmental cues act through hormones with the result that the organisms breed at favourable times of year: favourable for

13

the plant because it is the end of the growing season and food can be stored in the seeds; favourable for the animals since the young are not exposed to extreme cold and start to feed at a time when plenty of food is available.

In the British Isles, general observation will have shown you that the majority of plants grow rapidly in spring (mid-March to June), flower and produce seeds in summer (July to September) and either lose their leaves in the autumn and remain leafless until the following spring, or die, leaving seeds that overwinter to continue the species. There are, of course, exceptions—evergreen trees, plants that overwinter as roots or bulbs, plants that flower in mid-winter, and so on. The typical pattern of growth, flowering and fruiting is such that plants are active when external conditions of temperature and light are favourable for photosynthesis and are dormant during the cold, dark days of winter. Refer to Unit 7 (Section 7.2) and to Galston, Chapter 5, to remind yourself about the physiological mechanisms by which plant activity is related to environmental changes.

annual cycle of plant activity

The annual cycle of growth and dormancy in plants imposes an annual rhythm on herbivorous animals in addition to possible direct effects of temperature and light. How do these animals respond?

herbivores

The general pattern is that herbivorous animals grow in spring and summer when plants are growing. Many have annual life cycles, completing their growth in a few weeks and spending the rest of the year as resting stages such as the eggs and pupae of insects. Many invertebrates have life histories shorter than a year; they pass through several generations in the summer and overwinter as eggs, pupae or larvae of a winter generation.

Herbivorous mammals typically bear young in spring or early summer. These young and the adults feed through the summer and lay down stores of fat which are used up during the winter when food is scarce. Some small mammals, such as woodmice and squirrels, lay up stores of nuts and fruit. A few British mammals, such as hedgehogs, 'hibernate' (Fig. 7), that is, they fall into a 'winter sleep' when their body temperature is reduced. Breathing becomes slow and irregular and the heart beat slows; the metabolism is reduced to less than five per cent of normal. Even at this low metabolic rate, fat reserves are used up by the end of the winter.

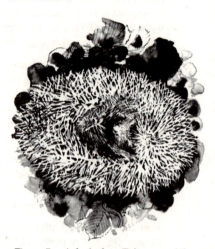

Figure 7 *A hedgehog* Erinaceus *hibernating.*

The cycle of annual abundance of herbivorous invertebrates, especially of insects, directly affects predators. In Britain, many birds have patterns of growth and reproduction that involve nesting and egg-laying in spring. The eggs hatch when actively growing insects, such as caterpillars, are very numerous and the parent birds spend the long daylight hours of May and June collecting food for their fast-growing young. Birds that are plant-feeders as adults, such as finches, commonly feed their young on insects; the diet changes when the young grow up. Like the mammals, birds store fat if they find sufficient food. Many small birds starve to death during winter when food is scarce. Many birds avoid wintry conditions by migrating south at the end of summer, returning north again the following spring; their long journeys expose them to many other hazards. The migratory habit has evolved in several different families of birds so there must be, on balance, a selective advantage for these species to brave the perils of migration rather than endure the privations of winter.

predators

From this very brief account of selected groups of animals, it is clear that spring and summer are periods of rapid growth and of reproduction in contrast to winter, when food is scarce. Animals survive winter conditions:

winter

(a)   by overwintering in a state which does not need food—as eggs or pupae or in hibernation,

(b)   by reducing the level of activity and consuming reserves of body fat or stored food but not becoming quiescent,

(c)   by migrating to places where food is available and conditions are less extreme.

There are many physiological problems associated with these life patterns; to quote a few:

(a)   How are the reproductive cycles of the animals (mammals, birds, insects) timed and adjusted to the annual cycle of climatic change and plant growth?

14

(b)   How is 'overwintering' controlled? How is the time of hatching of eggs or emergence of adults from pupae determined in spring? What factors are concerned with the beginning and end of hibernation?

(c)   How does the body 'switch' from a high level of activity and a régime where excess of food is available and is being transformed into fat reserves to a low level of activity and a régime where little food is eaten and fat stores are utilized and depleted?

(d)   What factors initiate and direct the migrations of birds (and of other animals that migrate, including mammals and insects) both southward in autumn and northward in spring?

You have read about some of these problems already in this Course. In Unit 8 you studied the reproductive cycle of mammals and the complex balance of hormones through which it is controlled; in Unit 9 you read about the control of metabolism.

ITQ 6   Briefly compare how flowering in chrysanthemums and the reproductive cycles of female sheep are related to annual climatic cycles. (Refer to Galston,* Chapter 5, and to Unit 8, if necessary.)

chrysanthemums and sheep

Read the answer to ITQ 6.

Observations of birds have shown that their reproductive cycles also are controlled through pituitary and gonadal hormones and related to changes in day-length. Initiation of migratory movements, also, appears to depend on changes in day-length and to be associated closely with reproductive development in spring.

What about insects? The dormant state in winter is an example of 'diapause', defined as a condition when developmental processes are arrested and metabolism falls to a very low level (note the similarity to hibernation). Insects may enter diapause at different stages of their life histories: as a developing embryo in the egg or as a larva about to pupate or as a pupa or adult. For any species, diapause occurs regularly only in one particular stage; many insects do not enter diapause but may show a reduced level of metabolism and slowed development. Various experiments have demonstrated that diapause is probably initiated and terminated by the action of hormones, but the details vary from species to species. Take the pupa of the silk-moth *Cecropia* as an example: this enters diapause in autumn and the moth emerges in the following spring. Pupae kept warm through the winter remain in diapause indefinitely, but if pupae are chilled to about 5 °C for a few days and then returned to warm conditions (20 to 25 °C), the diapause is broken and adult moths soon emerge. Williams[1] showed that transplanting a brain from a chilled pupa to a pupa which had been kept warm resulted in that pupa breaking diapause. However, the implanted chilled brain is only effective if the host pupa has an intact prothoracic gland *or* if a prothoracic gland is also implanted. Thus it seems that a hormone diffuses from the brain and affects the prothoracic gland from which a hormone diffuses to end diapause. One of the first signs of the end of diapause is the synthesis of the respiratory enzyme cytochrome oxidase; another is the appearance of the enzyme choline-esterase in the brain coupled with detectable electrical activity there.

diapause

ITQ 7   Compare diapause in insects with delayed implantation in mammals (refer back to Unit 8, if necessary).

ITQ 8   Compare the ending of diapause in insects with the initiation of germination in seeds.

Read the answers to ITQ 7 and 8,

So plants and animals may use similar environmental cues. The result is that their cycles of growth, feeding and abundance appear closely synchronized. In

* *A. W. Galston (1964) The Life of the Green Plant, 2nd ed. (Foundation of Modern Biology Series), Prentice-Hall.*

15

spring and early summer, plants are available as food for insects and insects as food for birds because all are responding to changes in day length or in temperature or in both.

11.4 Coupled Physiological Evolution in Unrelated Groups of Organisms

Study comment

Three types of food-web interrelationship are studied; first, some physiological adaptations in plants, which make them unpalatable or poisonous, have been matched by physiological adaptations in herbivorous insects that eat them; secondly, rabbit fleas have evolved so that their reproductive cycles are dependent on hormonal changes in their hosts; thirdly, well-adapted internal parasites and their hosts are mutually adapted physiologically. If short of time, you could omit Sections 11.4.1 and 11.4.3; you are advised to read Section 11.4.2 since it revises material from Units 8 and 9.

Interactions between unrelated species of organisms may be of several different types that can be summarized loosely as:

(a) Food-web interrelationships; these include predator–prey and parasite-host interactions.

(b) Shelter interrelationships; these include such situations as the presence of certain types of tree allowing certain birds to breed in an area, the presence of plants giving shelter to animals in streams and the presence of certain molluscs providing shells used later by other animals such as hermit crabs.

(c) Conditioning interrelationships; organisms 'condition' (change) the environment simply by living in it and the changed environment may then be suitable for organisms that could not live in it before or it may become unsuitable for other organisms. This type of change underlies 'ecological succession' (refer back to S100, Unit 20); a discipline called (in USA) 'allelochemics'[2] is emerging as the study of chemical substances produced by organisms, and part of its field covers 'conditioning'.

Here we study the physiological implications of interactions with three examples of food-web interrelationships.

11.4.1 Plants and herbivorous insects

Food-webs depend on plants performing photosynthesis and being eaten by animals. There are very large numbers of herbivorous species of animal actively feeding on living plants, yet green plants are common and conspicuous in most terrestrial environments. This observation implies that many herbivores are not limited in abundance by their food supply but by other factors that reduce population increase, such as predators. However, there is another explanation: that not all plants are palatable as food for animals, either all the time or part of the time. Insects include more species of animals than any other group (Subclass, Class or Phylum); many insect species are herbivorous and many herbivorous insects are highly specific in their feeding habits, confining themselves to one species of plant or a limited number of plant species. Some of these insect species are pests of plants useful to man, so there has been an economic motive for much research on plant-eating insects.

Caterpillars of many species of moth feed on oak leaves in spring (Fig. 8) and grow fast (refer to S100, Unit 20, for examples) but there are very few species of caterpillars feeding on oak leaves after late May and these grow slowly—have the leaves changed?

There is an increase in tannin content from about 0·7 per cent of the dry weight in April to about 5·5 per cent of the dry weight in September and the type of tannin changes from hydrolysable tannins in spring to condensed tannins in summer and autumn. Feeny[3] fed groups of winter moth caterpillars, some on fresh oak leaves collected in May and some on an artificial diet with no tannin

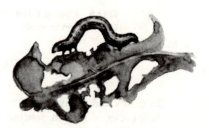

Figure 8 Winter moth caterpillar on an oak leaf.

in it; the two groups showed very similar rates of growth and turned into pupae of similar weights. The artificial diet was modified by substitution of some oak leaf tannin (extracted from leaves gathered in September) for some of the cellulose (which is probably not digested by these caterpillars). Caterpillars fed on modified diets turned into pupae that were markedly lighter than those fed on the original diet; with only 1 per cent of tannin per dry weight of the diet, the reduction of pupal weights was statistically significant.

Condensed tannins are laid down after the leaves have stopped growing; they bind proteins into indigestible complexes, that inhibit growth of caterpillars and of vertebrates. Tannins also inhibit the growth of fungi and multiplication of viruses; thus they protect the oak against a wide variety of organisms that could damage the tree either by destroying its photosynthetic apparatus or in other ways.

Tannins are just one example of substances produced by plants that act as defences against herbivorous animals; other such substances are the nicotine in tobacco plants and digitoxin (yielding digitalis) in foxgloves, both of which have deleterious physiological effects on animals that eat them (both affect heart function in mammals—see Unit 5). Plant metabolism may result in some waste substances; occasional mutants may produce substances unpalatable to animals. If there is no adverse effect on the plant, the better survival of the unpalatable plants may result in the mutant becoming the 'wild type'.

Provided that the production of the noxious substance is not too great a drain on metabolism, there is likely to be selection favouring individual plants with higher concentrations of the substance. As a result of adaptive radiation, it is likely that groups of related species will evolve with similar protective chemical substances. One example of this is the dicotyledonous family Cruciferae (wallflowers, cabbages) whose species are specialists in production of mustard oils and their glycosides.

Defensive substances in plants mean that many herbivorous animals will not (cannot) eat them. But herbivorous animals also undergo mutation and any mutant that can eat a noxious plant is faced with much less competition than a form feeding on a palatable plant. So it is not surprising that, for each group of noxious plants, there are herbivorous insects that feed on them; cabbage white butterfly caterpillars (Fig. 9), mustard beetles and cabbage aphids feed on cruciferous leaves. A further twist to the story is the evolution of adaptive behaviour of these insects which find their food plants by responding to the odour of mustard oils; the chemical defence system of the plant now acts as an attractant to its specialized herbivores. The garden nasturtium *Tropaeolum* produces mustard oils chemically similar to those of Cruciferae; although *Tropaeolum* belongs to a quite different family of angiosperms (Tropaeolaceae), many insects that attack cruciferous plants also attack it.

Herbivorous species that have become adapted to feed on poisonous plants may attain a further advantage if the poison persists in their bodies and renders them poisonous to possible predators. A group of American plants called 'milkweeds' of the family Asclepiadaceae contain *cardiac glycosides* (like digitoxin) that affect vertebrate hearts. Several insect species that feed on milkweed, including a grasshopper[4] and caterpillars of the monarch butterfly[5] (see Fig. 10) retain some of the toxic substances, discarding others; these insects are very distasteful to birds (they are also brightly coloured, conspicuous insects, examples of 'warning coloration').

Remarkable from the point of view of respiratory biochemistry are plants and insects that are tolerant to HCN. HCN inhibits the cytochrome system and is lethal in minute quantities to most organisms. Some plants produce *cyanogenic glycosides*; these hydrolyse to release HCN. The kernels of almonds, peach and related plants (family Rosaceae) contain amygdalin that hydrolyses to yield benzaldehyde (the characteristic smell of almonds) and HCN. Bird's foot trefoil plants (family Leguminosae) may contain quite high concentrations of HCN in spring and none in the autumn; plants from different localities differ in amounts present. The trefoil plants are able to survive and grow with quite high concentrations; they are avoided by rabbits and other mammalian herbivores. The common blue butterfly (Fig. 11) feeds as a caterpillar on bird's foot trefoil[6]; caterpillars can grow as well on plants with HCN as on those that have none. Larvae of the brightly coloured Burnet moth (see Fig. 12) also feed on bird's foot

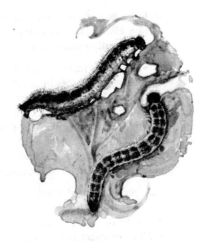

Figure 9 *Cabbage white caterpillars on a cabbage leaf.*

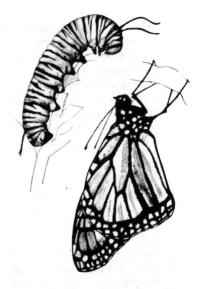

Figure 10 *Monarch butterfly and caterpillar.*

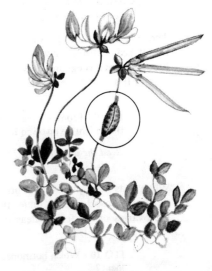

Figure 11 *Common blue caterpillar on a bird's foot trefoil plant.*

trefoil[7], as well as other species of trefoil and clover. All stages of this moth release HCN when body tissues are crushed; they are poisonous to predators[8] (this is another example of 'warning coloration').

A very subtle form of defence by plants is the production of substances that operate as hormones in insects; several gymnosperm species are now known to produce substantial amounts of substances identical with insect hormones and also some related chemical substances that are even more potent. This was first noticed in experiments with *Cecropia* (silk moth) where paper was ingested by caterpillars and caused acceleration of metamorphosis with consequent death. Eventually the 'paper factor' was traced back to the balsam fir, used very commonly in paper manufacture.

The production of similar chemical compounds by diverse organisms should not surprise you since the basic biochemistry of cells is very similar in the majority of living organisms. Nevertheless, it is remarkable that some plants synthesize insect hormones, that similar cardiac glycosides occur in plants and as toad venoms (toads are carnivores) that onions and skunks both produce evil-smelling *mercaptans*—and so on.

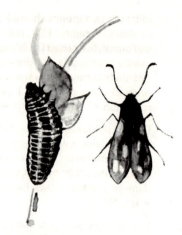

Figure 12   Six-spot Burnet moth and its caterpillar.

11.4.2   Rabbits and rabbit fleas[9, 10]

When myxomatosis reached Britain and killed more than eighty million rabbits in two years, attention was focused on the rabbit flea *Spilopsyllus cuniculi* because it transmitted the virus that caused the disease from one rabbit to another. For accounts of myxomatosis in Australia and Britain, see S100, Units 19 and 20. Attempts were made to rear rabbit fleas in laboratory conditions using techniques that are successful with the rat flea (which transmits bubonic plague) but, surprisingly, the fleas would not breed although they lived for months on tame rabbits. At the same time, eggs and larvae were found in the nests of wild rabbits—what was lacking in the laboratory?

myxomatosis

The life history of the flea is: eggs are laid in burrows where young 'nestling' rabbits live until ready to emerge to feed on plants. The eggs hatch into larvae that feed mainly on dried blood that has passed through the gut of adult fleas, been defaecated and added to the debris in the nest. The egg, larval and pupal stages (see Fig. 13) are completed in about 30 days, by which time the young rabbits have left the nest. Freshly emerged rabbit fleas seek hosts; they tend to gather on the rabbit's muzzle and cheeks, feeding at the base of the whiskers. Later, they move to the ears and fix themselves to the skin where groups of 10 to 150 individuals may be found through the spring and summer; in cold weather, they shift to sites where there is long fur. These fleas are feeding on rabbit blood and they defaecate about twice every hour. Male and female fleas may live side-by-side but on solitary rabbits they do not copulate and the eggs of the female do not mature. Fleas may transfer themselves to other rabbits that come into close contact with their host; they tend to gather in large numbers on pregnant does (females)—and this observation provided a clue to the factors controlling reproduction of rabbit fleas.

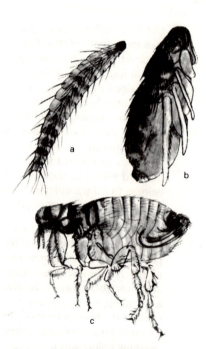

The first breakthrough was the demonstration that the ovaries of the female rabbit flea matured only on pregnant does, suggesting that some difference in blood between pregnant does and all other rabbits triggered off ovarian maturation in fleas. At once attention was focused on hormones.

Figure 13   The rabbit flea Spilopsyllus cuniculi: (a) *larva*; (b) *pupa*; (c) *adult*.

> **ITQ 9**   From information given in Units 8 and 9, suggest rabbit hormones that might be involved in this stimulation of ovarian development in the flea.
>
> *Read the answer to ITQ 9.*

When fleas were put on to a normal female rabbit which was then mated to a sterilized (vasectomized) male, the doe ovulated and became pseudopregnant; the ovaries of the female fleas matured on the fourteenth day.

> **ITQ 10**   Which hormones are eliminated as possible triggers by this experiment?
>
> *Read the answer to ITQ 10.*

18

Hormones concerned with pregnancy in the rabbit induce maturation of ovaries of female fleas, as demonstrated in the experiment above. Male fleas also showed changes. The next experiment was to inject a castrated buck (male rabbit) with extract of anterior pituitary; female fleas feeding on this buck developed mature ovaries and laid eggs (that were sterile because they had not been fertilized).

fleas and hormones

ITQ 11 Does this experiment mean that attention must now be directed only at the anterior pituitary and its hormones?

ITQ 12 Which hormones now remain for further investigation?

Read the answers to ITQs 11 and 12.

A typical later experiment was to inject luteinizing hormone (LH) into an ovariectomized doe and observe what happened to the fleas.

ITQ 13 What would be indicated by: (a) maturation of flea ovaries; (b) no change in flea ovaries?

Read the answer to ITQ 13.

As a result of a series of similar experiments, Rothschild and Ford[10] showed that the most effective hormones are corticosteroids produced by the adrenal glands under control of ACTH from the pituitary gland. Less effective were oestradiol and thyroxin; fleas can mature on thyroidectomized rabbits so thyroxin clearly is not essential even though it is effective in large doses.

fleas' maturation

Fleas were sprayed with hormone solutions, then placed on castrated buck rabbits. Fleas sprayed with corticosteroids, especially hydrocortisone (and to a lesser extent, with oestrogens) matured and laid eggs, remaining mature for long periods.

ITQ 14 From this would you conclude: (a) that rabbit hormones affect fleas as a result of their effect on rabbit metabolism, or (b) that rabbit hormones affect fleas directly?

Read the answer to ITQ 14.

When fleas mature there are changes in other parts of the body as well as maturation of sperm and ova. The gut enlarges and feeding rate of both sexes increases; mature males defaecate every four minutes, mature females once a minute.

ITQ 15 Suggest how this increased rate of defaecation is of importance for breeding success of fleas.

Read the answer to ITQ 15.

Fleas do not normally pair on pregnant does; any eggs laid on these are sterile because they are not fertilized. Shortly after the doe has produced her young (see Fig. 14), the fleas leave her ears and move on to her face; as she tends the young, the fleas move on to them and spread out, many settling on the back and flanks. At this stage, the fleas pair; both sexes feed while pairing. The female fleas leave the bodies of the young rabbits and lay their eggs in the nest; these eggs hatch and pass through larval and pupal stages in about 30 days. When her young are two to three weeks old, the fleas return to the doe even though they still have sperm and eggs ready to shed. Once back on the doe, the fleas change to a 'spent' state with gonads resembling those of immature fleas; the eggs are resorbed, the gut shrinks and so on. If the doe becomes pregnant again, then the fleas may mature again and move on to the new litter, pair and produce more fertilized eggs.

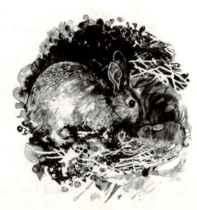

Figure 14 *Rabbit female with nestlings, about 19 days old, in their burrow.*

The fleas' reproductive cycle in the nest has been investigated and related to hormones in the hosts. Let us take the events described above in order:

19

Why do fleas leave the doe for the young? Perhaps because of an increase in the level of corticosteroids in the doe; injection of hydrocortisone at a low level induces fleas to attach closely to the host but a higher level makes them restless.

Why do the fleas copulate on the newly born young? The corticosteroid level is high in these nestlings; this may explain the rapid feeding but it does not explain pairing since, when older nestlings are injected with corticosteroids, this does not induce pairing. It seems that the female flea feeding on young nestlings becomes receptive to the male and stimulates him to copulate, possibly by releasing an attractive substance (a pheromone). Female fleas are ready to pair after a very short time on a new-born rabbit. When older nestlings were injected with pituitary growth hormone, fleas put on to them started to pair within two hours of the females starting to feed. The results are not so clear with rabbits eight weeks old; perhaps other stimulatory factors are required or perhaps inhibitory factors appear in older rabbits.

fleas' copulation

Why do the fleas go back to the doe? Perhaps there is some change in the relative hormone levels of mother and young; this has not been investigated fully.

When the fleas return to the doe, their gonads regress and their feeding activity falls off: how is this brought about? Simply starving fleas does not lead to such rapid regression of gonads as happens on the doe rabbit though the fall in food intake gradually has effects. So what about hormones?

regression of flea gonads

The doe at this stage is lactating and returning to a pro-oestrous state. Hormones circulating at this stage include LH and progesterone. There is a decrease in circulating corticosteroids but in experimental situations, fleas respond slowly by reduced feeding to change in level of these; they do not display the rapid regression observed in nature.

Buck rabbits were injected regularly with hydrocortisone; fleas on these rabbits showed maturation of gonads and increased defaecation. When progesterone was injected in addition to the hydrocortisone, defaecation became less frequent and eggs were resorbed; within two weeks, the fleas resembled normal 'spent' fleas. When injections of progesterone were stopped but those of hydrocortisone continued, the fleas were mature again within two weeks. Similar experiments with luteinizing hormone (LH) instead of progesterone gave similar results; fleas became 'spent' within a few days of injection of LH and became mature once more a few days after the injections of LH stopped.

One final question: how do the rabbit hormones act on the rabbit flea: do they affect the insect's gonads directly or do they influence the secretion of the flea's own hormones? Probably the rabbit hormones affect the balance between the flea's own hormones, but this has not been fully investigated. Certainly the larva of the flea behaves like other insect larvae and presumably has the full complement of hormones.

flea hormones

ITQ 16   Now suggest why the attempts to rear rabbit fleas in the laboratory, described in the first paragraph of this Section, were unsuccessful.

Read the answer to ITQ 16.

Rabbits are specialized mammals. The underground nesting habit provides an ideal protected environment for the development of flea larvae but rabbit nestlings grow fast so the nest is occupied for a limited period only. The rabbit flea is remarkable for its very short breeding period which is synchronized very accurately with that of an individual rabbit; this is possible because the adult flea responds to hormones circulating in the blood of the rabbit on which it feeds. No other species of flea is known to do this, though it is possible that bat fleas may have interesting physiological specializations. Clearly physiological evolution of the rabbit flea has proceeded in a direction that has adapted the insect extraordinarily well to the habits of its mammalian host.

11.4.3   Internal parasites and their hosts

In this type of relationship, the two species are in a continuous state of intimate mutual contact, so both the parasite and the host influence each other in various ways. This interaction involves a number of physiological adjustments, the details varying with the location of the parasite within the body, whether in the gut, the blood system, the body cavity or the muscles. The influence exerted by the parasite on the host may be the result of: mechanical damage; withdrawal from the host of certain essential substances normally required for the host's correct metabolism; the release of toxic substances; increasing the susceptibility of the host to other invading pathogenic organisms. Host reactions directed towards the parasite involve cell and tissue reactions and humoral reactions. The most common result of the former is the inflammation of host tissue which often results in the formation of a capsule around the parasite, thus breaking its contact with the host. Humoral reactions of the host are closely connected with the phenomenon of immunity, i.e. the production of antibodies which may result in various degrees of resistance towards the present or subsequent parasitic infection.

A parasite finds within its host two physiological 'environments', one being a 'nutritional environment', where various nutrient substances are available to it, the other an 'inhibitory environment', where mechanisms set up by the host tend to hinder the development of the parasite. Usually, the parasite's existence results from a balance between these two 'environments'. If the parasite finds in the host the correct nutrients, amino acids, vitamins, growth factors, etc., while inhibitory factors such as humoral and cellular defence mechanisms are virtually absent, then it thrives. This often happens when a parasite species attacks a new host species or a population of the host species that has not been in contact with this parasite before, e.g. sleeping sickness (caused by a protozoan *Trypanosoma*) killed many thousands of people in Uganda in the 1920s because the species concerned had arrived from further south and was new to that district. In many host-parasite interactions the two environments tend to balance each other to a certain extent so that the relationship is a reasonably harmonious one.

host environments

The adaptation of a parasite to its host and that of the host to its parasites develop gradually over a period of time. Some parasites become highly specific to one species of host, this representing a certain stage in the evolution of that relationship. Such specificity is not always stable; it is subject to modifications in different directions during the process of evolution and this is under the influence of various environmental factors. For instance, chemical and cellular defences of the host are clearly subject to selection, those developing the most successful defence being selected in an evolutionary sense because those hosts with fewest parasites are likely to have more food reserves to devote to reproduction (and hence to perpetuation of the species). However, the evolution of a parasitic species should progress mainly in parallel with that of its host, usually with just a small delay in physiological changes of the parasite following those of the host.

11.5 Physiological Mechanisms as Evidence for Phylogeny

Study comment

You are asked to work through all the physiological functions of animals, discussed in earlier Units, and to consider how differences in physiology tie up with ideas about the evolution of animal groups as discussed in Unit 1. The answers form summaries of the Units from this particular point of view so you are advised to read them; the final two paragraphs sum up this Section.

In *The Origin of Species* Charles Darwin presented evidence to support the theory that all living organisms have descended from ancestors unlike themselves as a result of natural selection acting upon variation. Almost all his examples were structural modifications. Until recently, anatomical observations were the main foundation on which organisms were grouped into hierarchies of taxa to form natural systems of classification; the usefulness of such systems was discussed in Units 1 and 3 which also included discussion of the principal groups of animals and plants. Now that we have reached the end of this short course on comparative physiology, it seems a fitting time to enquire whether knowledge of physiological mechanisms has contributed to the study of phylogeny.

Of the five Kingdoms of living organisms, we have been concerned with two only, the Plant and Animal Kingdoms. In Unit 1, Table 1, the principal difference between these is shown as the presence or absence of green plastids and, in Section 11.2, the consequences of this difference in nutritional ability are shown to include most of the striking anatomical and behavioural differences between plants and animals. Thus a fundamental physiological difference underlies the separate evolution of these two Kingdoms.

plants and animals

Your study of plant physiology has been confined almost entirely to angiosperms, the fairly homogeneous group which includes the majority of modern plant species. You are not really in a position to consider whether study of physiological mechanisms can contribute to evolutionary theories about plants; we shall therefore confine the discussion in this section to the Animal Kingdom.

Your study of animal physiology has been concentrated on two phyla: Chordata and Arthropoda; but it has included Annelida and Mollusca and occasional reference to members of other phyla. Within the phylum Chordata, attention has been concentrated on mammals and on teleost fishes, but other fishes, amphibians, reptiles and birds have received occasional mention. Within the Arthropoda, the emphasis has been on insects and crustaceans. In Unit 1, Section 1.5, two super-phyla were defined and a tentative evolutionary tree was constructed, based on anatomical features and structures basic to movement.

> Arrange the groups mentioned in this paragraph to show their relationship as suggested in Unit 1. Compare your 'tree' with that in Figure 15 (p. 24).

Are there fundamental physiological differences between the animals of the main branches of the tree in Figure 15? Try to answer this by working through the physiological functions discussed in Units 4, 5, 6, 8, 9 and 10. Write down your conclusions, then compare them with those given in Appendix I on p. 25.

From this survey of earlier Units there seems to emerge the conclusion that similar solutions to physiological problems are observed in species living under similar environmental stresses. An evolutionary series based on physiological studies would read like this:

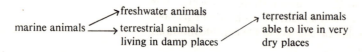

Insects and birds would qualify as the most highly evolved animals, with teleost fishes, some crustaceans and molluscs, and mammals in the middle grade. But it is not possible to believe that insects and birds really are more closely related to each other than birds are to mammals or insects are to crustaceans!

When the anatomical structures involved in physiological mechanisms are observed, it becomes clear that similar physiological mechanisms can occur in very different structures as, for example, the excretion of uric acid by the kidneys of birds and the Malpighian tubules of insects. Evolutionary lines based on comparison of structure make sense and are supported by study of fossil evidence. It seems that evolution by modification of inherited structures has been the general rule among animals. The cells within these structures have a certain amount of versatility, biochemically and at the organelle level, and this allows for the appearance of similar physiological solutions to environmental problems in unrelated or distantly related animals.

convergent evolution of physiological mechanisms

So our general conclusion must be that the study of comparative physiology contributes little to constructing phylogenetic trees at the level of phyla and classes; such phylogeny is better based on comparative anatomy and embryology. The differences which give phyla their distinctive characters are differences in structure—body cavity, segmentation, skeleton, ciliation and so on. Adaptive radiation within phyla is the result of adaptations of structure and also of physiological mechanisms; at the species level, physiological adaptations may be as important diagnostic features as the structural adaptations to which they are closely related. Physiological adaptations fit organisms to their environments; the degree to which such adaptations are possible must· depend on the degree to which the basic anatomy of a species (or genus or family) can vary and respond to selection. Why are there so few marine insects? Their basic anatomy, so wonderfully versatile under conditions of life on land or in freshwaters— even in highly saline waters—apparently has not allowed widespread adaptation to marine conditions. So we end, as we began the Course, by stressing that structure and function are initimately related; that one cannot be understood without some knowledge of the other; that organisms show adaptations to their environments and are best studied in relation to their whole way of life.

Summary

This Unit revises the earlier Units by setting the information in them into different frames of reference.

Eucaryotic cells all have many mechanisms in common; the principal contrast is between those cells with green plastids and those without (Section 11.1).

The possession of cells with green plastids, conferring the ability to perform photosynthesis, is the basis for very considerable differences between plants and animals, discussed in Section 11.2. These differences include degree of mobility, type of internal circulation, shape and size of body, reproduction, co-ordination and regulation.

Organisms live in environments with definite physical and chemical features that may vary regularly. Unrelated organisms show similar adaptations to environmental factors. Plants and animals have physiological mechanisms that often depend on similar environmental cues, as illustrated (Section 11.3) by study of annual cycles in the British Isles and the responses of plants, mammals, birds and insects.

Organisms of any species have contacts with organisms of other species. Sometimes there has been evolution of physiological mechanisms in one species that correlate with physiological mechanisms that have evolved in another, unrelated species. Such evolution is illustrated in Section 11.4 by study of: some interactions between plants that are poisonous or unpalatable and herbivorous insects that nevertheless feed on them; the dependence of reproduction in the rabbit flea on hormonal changes in its host; the mutual evolution between internal parasites and their hosts.

Evolution is an important theme that underlies the whole Course. Section 11.5 is a discussion of the relevance of comparative physiology to phylogenetic studies of animals. Physiological adaptations fit organisms to their environments and may be important diagnostic features at the species level. The distinctive differences between phyla, however, are differences in structure. There is considerable convergence in physiological mechanisms between unrelated organisms that live in similar environments.

References

1 C. M. Williams (1946) Brain hormones in Lepidopteran metamorphosis. *Biol. Bull.* **90**, pp. 234–43.
————— (1947) Roles of brain and prothoracic gland principles in Lepidoteran metamorphosis. *Biol. Bull.* **93**, pp. 89–98.
————— (1947) Brain and termination of pupal diapause *Anat. Rec.* **99**, p. 671.
————— (1952) Brain and prothoracic gland in insect metamorphosis. *Biol. Bull.* **103**, pp. 120–38.

2 R. H. Whittaker and P. P. Feeny (1971) Allelochemics: Chemical interactions between species. *Science*, **171**, pp. 757–70.

3 P. P. Feeny (1968) Effect of oak leaf tannins on larval growth of the winter moth *Operophtera brumata. J. Insect Physiology*, **14**, pp. 805–17.

4 J. von Euw, L. Fishelson, J. A. Parsons, T. Reichstein and Miriam Rothschild (1967) Cardenolides (heart poisons) in a grasshopper feeding on
   milkweeds. *Nature, London*, **214,** pp. 35–9.

5 T. Reichstein, J. von Euw, J. A. Parsons and Miriam Rothschild (1968)
   Heart poisons in the monarch butterfly. *Science*, **161,** pp. 861–6.

6 Charles Lane (assisted by Miriam Rothschild) (1962) Notes on the common
   blue (*Polyommatus icarus* (Rott.)) egg-laying and feeding on the cyanogenic
   strains of the bird's-foot trefoil (*Lotus corniculatus* L.) *Entomologists'
   Gazette*, **13,** pp. 112–16.

7 Charles Lane (assisted by Miriam Rothschild) (1959) A very toxic moth:
   the five-spot Burnet (*Zygaena trifolii* Esp.) *Entomologists' Monthly Magazine*,
   94, pp. 93–4.

8 David A. Jones, John Parsons and Miriam Rothschild (1962) Release
   of hydrocyanic acid from crushed tissues of all stages in the life-cycle of
   species of the Zygaeninae (Lepidoptera). *Nature, London*, **193,** pp. 52–3.

9 Miriam Rothschild (1965) The rabbit flea and hormones. *Endeavour*, **24,**
   pp. 162–8.

10 Miriam Rothschild and Bob Ford (1966) Hormones of the vertebrate host
   controlling ovarian regression and copulation of the rabbit flea. *Nature,
   London*, **211,** pp. 261–6.

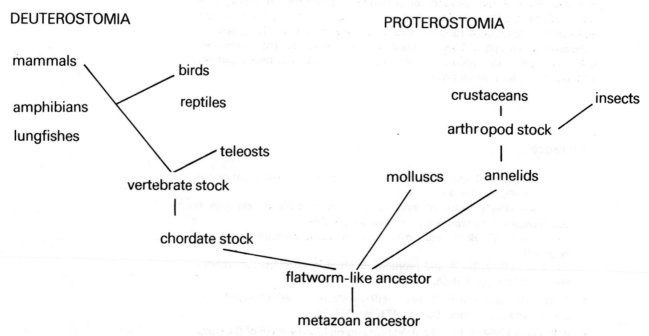

Figure 15 *Phylogenetic 'tree'.*

Appendix I

Diversity of Physiological Functions among Animals discussed in Units 4, 5, 6, 8, 9 and 10

Nutrition (*Unit 4*)

The food eaten by animals and their methods of capturing it are very varied but seem more obviously related to the habitats and sizes of the animals than to their systematic position. Ciliary microphagous feeding is displayed by some annelids, molluscs and chordates (e.g. *Amphioxus*); some crustaceans are microphagous feeders but have no cilia, depending instead on setae on their appendages. Here is an interesting difference at the level of *cell organelles* between members of the phylum Arthropoda, which lack motile cilia, and members of the other phyla you have studied all of which have some ciliated cells in their bodies. The mechanisms for microphagous feeding are consequently different in arthropods from those of the other phyla. Macrophagous feeders are found in all the phyla studied, with similar adaptations differing in detail. Digestive mechanisms, ranging from intracellular to extracellular types, are basically similar in all, but with differences in details; the presence of symbionts in the guts of insects that feed on wood and mammals that eat grass is a striking example of convergence. Molluscs are exceptional in their ability to digest wood and cellulose with their own xylases and cellulases.

Circulation of the blood (*Unit 5*)

Two contrasted types of circulation exist: open (as in gastropod molluscs and arthropods); closed (as in annelids, cephalopod molluscs and vertebrates). Open systems are associated with haemocoelic body cavities. The closed systems of annelids and vertebrates are associated with coelomic main body cavities but cephalopods have achieved a closed system by constricting the haemocoel while retaining a restricted coelom. The general trend, from contractile vessels in more primitive animals to a contractile organ, the heart, in more advanced animals can be illustrated by examples drawn from Proterostomes and from Deuterostomes; even the evolution of double circulations can be illustrated by examples drawn from molluscs and from vertebrates, with the final patterns different in structure though similar in physiological function.

Respiratory mechanisms (*Unit 6*)

Aquatic animals typically exchange gases in solution whereas terrestrial animals 'breathe' air; larger animals in both environments usually have respiratory organs called 'gills' in water and 'lungs' on land. But there is a notable exception: the insects (and some other arthropod groups) have a tracheal system that is unique to the phylum Arthropoda; its evolution probably became possible with the evolution of an exoskeleton based on chitin. Chitin is produced by many phyla of animals but arthropods mix it with tanned proteins or with calcium salts and produce a variety of exoskeletons combining strength with plasticity (at joints) and general waterproofing with local permeability. The presence of tracheae means that the blood of most insects has no respiratory function and that most insects have no respiratory pigment. This contrasts with vertebrates, almost all of which have haemoglobin as respiratory pigment, and molluscs and crustaceans, which typically have haemocyanin.

Hormones and reproduction (*Unit 8*)

Since you have studied this topic almost entirely in mammals, you will not be able to make useful comparisons. Hormones are involved in reproductive cycles of insects; many invertebrates have not been investigated at all.

Hormones and homeostasis (*Unit 9*)

Again, most of your information comes from studies of mammals and you will not be able to compare them with animals of other phyla.

Osmo-regulation and excretion (*Unit 10*)

For these functions you should have enough information for some interesting tentative conclusions. Claude Bernard's famous statement about the constancy of the internal environment seems to apply to most metazoans. For many marine species, sea water is an adequate substitute for their body fluids which are similar to seawater in ionic constitution and total osmotic pressure; this observation supports the theory that metazoans evolved in the sea as aggregates of cells bathed in sea water. The sea is still the habitat for the majority of animal species *excluding* the insects (half the Animal Kingdom!) Animals living in freshwaters have body fluids of higher osmotic pressure than the water round them so are in constant danger of dilution of their internal environment and often in danger of swelling up and bursting as water floods in. External waterproofing and the presence of 'kidneys' with salt-absorbing tubules are characteristic of freshwater molluscs*, vertebrates and crustaceans. Fully terrestrial animals are in danger of dehydration and concentration of body fluids; complete water-proofing is not possible because exchange of respiratory gases appears to require an epithelium that is permeable and damp (Unit 6). The convergent and indepen-dent evolution of physiological devices that reduce water loss is the solution to this problem in vertebrates, molluscs*, crustaceans and insects.

The need for elimination of excess nitrogenous compounds in animals has already been mentined (Section 11.2.6). Basically, ammonia is the simplest nitrogenous compound excreted and probably involves the lowest metabolic 'cost' to produce, but it must be eliminated either by diffusion into water or as a dilute solution, which involves loss of much water at the same time. Urea is a more sophisticated excretory compound but it also must be eliminated as a dilute solution. Terrestrial animals that live in dry places characteristically produce uric acid (or a related purine) and eliminate it in a semi-solid state with little water; this solution to the problem of water conservation is found in vertebrates (birds and some reptiles), molluscs (snails), crustaceans (some woodlice) and insects. The structures in which the uric acid is produced are very different in these groups but there is clear physiological convergence (and the biochemical mechanisms are similar).

---

* *Molluscs were not mentioned in Unit 10, but fit into the general pattern described there.*

Self-assessment Questions

SAQ 1 (*Objective 2*) Taking angiosperms as typical plants and mammals as typical animals, consider each of the attributes listed below—decide for each one whether it is typical of plants only, typical of animals only, typical of plants and animals or not typical of either.

Mark: P for typical of plants only.

A for typical of animals only.

B for typical of both plants and animals.

N for not typical of either plants or animals.

1 Ability to synthesize sugar and amino acids from water, carbon dioxide and salts.

2 Ability to derive energy from activity by enzymic breakdown of sugars.

3 Ability to ingest other organisms.

4 Ability to grow in volume.

5 Possession of a diffuse shape.

6 Ability to move from place to place.

7 Possession of a circulatory system with a pumping organ.

8 Possession of supporting tissue that also is part of the circulatory system.

9 Possession of a compact shape.

10 Ability to show differential growth.

11 Possession of roots in the ground.

12 Possession of a circulation that depends on water potential.

13 Life history includes alternation of generations.

14 Cells within organism can communicate rapidly with others at a distance via specialized cells.

15 Ability to survive temperatures close to 100 °C.

16 Cells within organism can influence others at a distance via chemical substances.

17 Majority of body cells are diploid.

18 Ability to survive without oxygen for long periods of time.

19 Sensitivity to incident light.

20 Ability to form social groups.

SAQ 2 (*Objective 5*) Consider the following statements about aposematic caterpillars (caterpillars which have warning coloration):

(a) All aposematic caterpillars derive their repellent properties directly from their food plants.

(b) Those aposematic caterpillars that specialize in feeding on one group of closely related plants derive their repellent qualities from their food plants.

(c) Those aposematic caterpillars that can feed on a wide variety of plants produce poisonous or repellent substances independently of any that occur in their food plants.

(1) Are the three statements (a), (b) and (c) consistent with each other?

(2) If the three statements are not consistent with each other, are two of them consistent with each other? If so, which two?

(3) From the information given in Section 11.4.1, decide whether each of the statements (a), (b) and (c) is or is not likely to be true. Try to support your conclusions by quoting examples from the text.

SAQ 3 (*Objectives 5 and 6*) The grasshopper *Poekilocercus bufonius* eats milkweeds but can also be reared on other plants. Adults and hoppers (nymphs) each have a bilobed poison gland. When irritated, the animals secrete a liquid which has a disagreeable smell and produces a prickling sensation when applied to the human tongue.

Consider the following results of analyses:

	Grasshoppers fed on:	
	milkweed (asclepiad plant)	composite plant (of daisy family)
Histamine content of poison gland secretion (measured as equivalent to content of wasp sting)	1 sting	1 sting
Cardiac glycoside content of poison gland secretion (measured as equivalent to lethal dose for cat)	1 dose	0·1 dose
Histamine content of haemolymph	0·001 sting	not known
Cardiac glycoside content of haemolymph	1 dose	not known

Consider whether each of the following statements (a) to (d) is *either* a warranted deduction from the information above *or* unwarranted because it clearly is not true *or* unwarranted because there is not enough information to warrant the deduction:

(a) The histamine in the poison gland secretion is derived from the diet.

(b) The histamine in the poison gland secretion is synthesized in the poison gland.

(c) The cardiac glycosides in the poison gland secretion are derived from the diet.

(d) The cardiac glycosides in the poison gland secretion are synthesized in the poison gland.

Further analyses revealed that there are two main cardiac glycosides in the secretions of grasshoppers fed on milkweed: calaction and calotropin (both have actions similar to digitalis). Consider the following results of analyses:

	Approximate concentration in mg per animal	
	Calactin	Calotropin
Secretion from adults fed on milkweed	0·2	0·2
Secretion from hoppers fed on milkweed	0·14	0·06
Secretion from hoppers fed on other plants but with parents that fed on milkweed	0·01	0·01
Secretion from hoppers fed on other plants and with parents that fed on other plants	0·002	0·001
Concentration in whole eggs of grasshoppers which fed on milkweed	0·01	0·01

27

Milkweed plants contain six or more cardiac glycosides: of these, *only* calactin and calotropin are found in the poison gland secretion.

From all the information presented, consider each of the following statements (e) to (j) and decide whether the statement is probably true *or* probably not true *or* whether it is impossible to judge whether the statement is true or untrue because of lack of essential evidence.

(e)   The calactin and calotropin in the poison gland secretion are derived from the diet.

(f)   The grasshopper is unable (at any stage) to synthesize either calactin or calotropin (except perhaps from precursors in milkweed).

(g)   The grasshopper probably selectively absorbs calactin and calotropin from its diet but does not absorb the other glycosides in milkweed.

(h)   The grasshopper probably absorbs all the glycosides in its diet but actively excretes all except calactin and calotropin.

(i)   the grasshopper probably absorbs all the glycosides in its diet but metabolizes all except calactin and calotropin.

(j)   The grasshopper probably absorbs all the glycosides in the diet and then converts all the others into either calactin or calotropin.

Answers to In-text Questions

ITQ 1 Pollen grains are spores which grow into the male gametophyte generation when they reach the stigma of a flower. The male gamete is a nucleus in the pollen tube; it fuses with the female nucleus (the nucleus of the ovule) and the zygote gives rise by division to the embryo in the seed. Pollen grains are waterproofed and may be distributed by the wind or through the agency of animals such as bees and butterflies (refer back to S100, Unit 21, to remind yourself about the co-adaptation of insects and flowers). Refer back to Unit 2 to remind yourself about the life histories of angiosperms.

ITQ 2 Both groups have internal fertilization; males have specialized intromittent organs (the penis in mammals). Sperm is transferred during copulation from the male into the female's reproductive tract; the ovum is fertilized inside the female. In mammals, the fertilized egg develops inside the female but, in insects, the egg is usually enclosed in a waterproofed shell and laid. It may develop at once or remain dormant for a period (see Section 11.3).

ITQ 3 Water provides more support than air; terrestrial organisms live in danger of dehydration yet respiratory surfaces must be kept moist. The groups of terrestrial animals with most species are the insects (arthropods) and vertebrates; both have skeletons (Unit 1). Terrestrial plants have supporting tissue (fibres and xylem, Unit 2). Terrestrial animals have external layers that are waterproofed (Units 6 and 10); terrestrial plants also have waterproofed epithelial cells (TV programme of Unit 2). Terrestrial animals lose water during respiration and excretion (Units 6 and 10); terrestrial plants lose water during transpiration and respiration (Units 2 and 3). Water and land environments also differ in degree of exposure to changes in temperature (more rapid on land) and light intensity (higher on land). At high altitudes the atmosphere becomes rarefied, while at great depths pressures become very high and there is no sunlight. In general, land environments are more stressful than aquatic ones to both plants and animals.

ITQ 4 Animals have fluids (blood or extracellular fluids) with osmotic pressures (due to salts and colloids and sugars) that are higher than that of fresh water. Since most aquatic animals have membranes that are permeable to water (respiratory surfaces, absorptive surfaces) there is a grave danger that water will enter the body, diluting the concentration of the body fluids. Animals that respire oxygen dissolved in water, through gills typically, have the rest of the body surface impermeable to water, reducing the intake; they have some type of 'kidney' that pumps out the excess water. Compare fishes with crustaceans: both excrete water through modified coelomoducts (Unit 10) in which there is a terminal bulb and a long tubule; fishes have an impermeable outer layer to the skin, crustaceans have an impermeable exoskeleton reinforced with calcium salts; both have 'gills' where gas exchange takes place and water can enter the body.

ITQ 5 Ammonia is very toxic and can be disposed of only in very dilute solution. Urea also must be disposed of in solution—although much less toxic than ammonia, it exerts an osmotic pressure so the solution cannot be very concentrated; thus animals living under very dry conditions would benefit from producing a nitrogenous compound that is insoluble (almost), solid or semi-solid and non-toxic. Birds and insects both produce uric acid as principal excretory product. (Refer back to Unit 10 to revise this material.)

ITQ 6 In sheep and in chrysanthemums, the onset of reproduction is demonstrably related to shortening day-length (photoperiod); some part of the organism is sensitive to day-length and hormones reach the gonads or flowerbuds and stimulate their maturation. But sheeps' responses depend on the length of the *light* period whereas chrysanthemums' responses depend on the length of the *dark* period. Probably in plants, red light affecting the reversible breakdown in the *leaves* of a pigment *phytochrome* is the principal stimulus promoting flowering in long-day plants but inhibiting flowering in short-day plants such as chrysanthemums; a hormone *florigen* is postulated, travelling in the *phloem* from leaves to flower buds and stimulating maturation of the buds. In sheep, light affects centres in the *hypothalamus* via pathways that are not fully defined; the hypothalamus produces *FSH/LH-RF* and this reaches the pituitary through a *portal system* and stimulates secretion of *FSH* and *LH*; increasing levels of these hormones in the *blood* cause follicular growth and *oestrogen* secretion and so the sheep comes into oestrous at the appropriate time. Note that in plants more is known about the receptor side of the mechanism than the effectors, whereas, in animals, much more is known about the effector side and little about the receptor sites and pathways.

Temperature effects are important in some plants (e.g. wheats and biennials that require vernalization) and in some animals —but you have not met any relevant information about sheep and chrysanthemums.

ITQ 7 If diapause occurs when the insect is a developing embryo in the egg, then this corresponds to the stage in the mammal life cycle when delayed implantation occurs and a blastocyst remains in the same stage of development, sometimes for several months. But there are contrasts in the mechanisms that end the two rest periods: in mammals, implantation finally occurs as a result of hormonal changes in the mother but the insect egg has already been laid by the mother so the resumed development of the embryo in it is a direct response to environmental triggering. Insect eggs resemble seeds in this respect (see the next answer).

ITQ 8 Seeds are a dormant stage in the lives of plants; there are inhibitors that ensure that dormancy continues through dry or cold periods and germination occurs when there is water available and at seasons when the seedlings are likely to survive. Temperature is an important stimulus, as it is also in insects. The need for chilling before diapause ends, in *Cecropia*, is paralleled by the need for vernalization by chilling of some plants.

ITQ 9 In pregnant does the corpus luteum is active and there is a high level of progesterone in the blood as well as some oestrogen; the pituitary secretes much LH. There are also changes in level of other pituitary hormones and of hormones of the adrenal glands (corticosteroids). Substances produced by the placenta or passing from the foetal rabbits through the placenta could be present in the maternal blood.

ITQ 10 It eliminates placental hormones and any substances diffusing from foetal rabbits.

ITQ 11 No, because these pituitary hormones have among their target organs some that produce hormones (e.g. gonads, adrenals, thyroid gland).

ITQ 12 The hormones actually produced by the anterior pituitary (including TSH, ACTH, FSH, LH, prolactin) *and* hormones produced by the target organs (including androgens, oestrogens, progesterone, thyroxin, corticosteriods).

ITQ 13 (a) If the ovaries matured, this would indicate that LH initiated flea maturation either directly or through some intermediate effect; (b) if the ovaries remained unchanged, then LH could be removed from the list of possible trigger mechanisms.

ITQ 14 The hormone solutions were sprayed on to the fleas so the probability is (b) that they affect the fleas directly. There is no evidence that these hormones found their way into the rabbit blood, so it is very unlikely that there was any change in rabbit metabolism, therefore (a) is almost certainly unjustified as a conclusion.

ITQ 15 Flea larvae feed on dried blood that has passed through the adult fleas. The increased rate of defaecation that precedes pairing and egg-laying means that plenty of food will be available when the eggs hatch.

ITQ 16 The fleas were kept on solitary rabbits of both sexes in the laboratory. Since the female rabbits did not become pregnant or produce young, there was no maturation of the rabbit flea gonads and therefore no new generations of fleas were reared although the adults lived for months.

Self-assessment Answers and Comments

SAQ 1 1: P, 2: B, 3: A, 4: B, 5: P, 6: A, 7: A, 8: P, 9: A, 10: B, 11: P, 12: P, 13: P, 14: A, 15: N, 16: B, 17: B, 18: N, 19: B, 20: A.

Most of these are easy to answer and are referred to in Section 11.2; 13 and 17 were discussed in Unit 2 where life histories of animals and plants were contrasted.

14 Refers to the nervous system and 16 to hormones.

15 No living cells can survive temperatures as high as this.

18 This is difficult to answer because, in theory, plants in sunlight can produce enough oxygen to sustain their respiratory needs during darkness. The oxygen may diffuse away leaving the plants suffering from lack of oxygen. Angiosperms are not anaerobic organisms, nor are mammals—hence N is probably the best answer.

19 Many parts of plants are sensitive to light. Mammals typically have eyes; other parts of their bodies may also be sensitive to light (e.g. skin).

SAQ 2

(1) Statements (a) and (c) conflict with each other.

(2) Statements (b) and (c) are consistent with each other; (b) is also consistent with (a) but is unnecessary if (a) is true.

(3) Since there is conflict between statements (a) and (c), it seems worth testing these first. The only real piece of evidence that you have in the text is the statement about Burnet moth caterpillars: 'all stages of this moth release HCN when body tissues are crushed'. Relate this to the four preceding sentences which state that Burnet caterpillars feed on trefoils and clovers including bird's foot trefoil and that some plants of this last species have much HCN (from cyanogenic glycosides) and some have none. You can draw from these sentences the conclusion that Burnet caterpillars produce HCN when crushed whether or not they have fed on plants containing cyanogenic glycosides. This implies that Burnet caterpillars can produce the poisonous HCN independently of whether it is present in the food plant; they produce HCN when fed on cyanogenic strains of bird's foot trefoil and also when fed on harmless clover. So these caterpillars, that feed on a range of plant species, seem to confirm statement (c). If this is so, then statement (a) is untrue.

You can infer from the comments on the insects that feed on milkweeds that Monarch caterpillars acquire their repellent properties from their food plants. If these insects are confined to eating milkweeds (as they are) then their existence is evidence in favour of statement (b).

In fact, our text is too vague for you to feel happy that statements (b) and (c) are generally true, but you should conclude that statement (a) is *not* true. Historically, statement (a) was the first to be made about poisonous caterpillars and it was modified as a result of later investigations of many distasteful insects, which now appear to fall into two groups corresponding to statements (b) and (c).

SAQ 3

(a) Not warranted—the information suggests strongly that histamine is synthesized in the poison gland.

(b) Warranted—there is very little histamine in the haemolymph supplying the gland.

(c) Warranted—there are similar amounts of glycosides in the haemolymph and in the gland when the insect is fed on milkweed. On a diet of composite plant, the glycoside content of the gland is very low.

(d) Not warranted—the glycoside content of secretions of insects fed on milkweed (known to contain these glycosides) is ten times that of insects fed on composites (which probably contain much less, if any).

(e), (f) Warranted. Grasshoppers fed on milkweed produce comparatively large amounts of these two glycosides in the poison gland secretion. It appears that some glycoside is passed into the eggs; grasshoppers that have not fed on milkweed may secrete small amounts of inherited glycosides, the amount decreasing in the next generation that is fed on plants without glycosides. Hoppers kept in cages eat material that includes dried secretion and so many acquire fresh supplies of glycoside in their diet.

(g), (h), (i), (j) None of these are warranted deductions from the information given. Grasshoppers ingest milkweed containing six or more glycosides and they secrete poison containing only two of these but you have no information as to the fate of the other four. Each of the four statements could be true; it may be that each statement is true of some glycosides and not of others but it is very unlikely that all four statements are true of any one glycoside. Further evidence is essential before you could accept or dismiss any of these statements.

31

COMPARATIVE PHYSIOLOGY